Obesity's Economic Impact: Estimating Lifetime Costs

Billy Lee

Abstract [

This examines the increased prevalence of obesity in the context of market

failure. In welfare economics, market failure is an important precondition for government

intervention. Obesity in the United States has risen dramatically in the last several

decades; over two thirds of American adults are overweight, and one third is obese.

Obesity is a risk factor for a wide range of health conditions, including heart disease,

diabetes, cancer, stroke, and osteoarthritis. In addition to the significant human costs,

there are economic ramifications to the sequelae of obesity, such as increased costs

associated with healthcare, disability and absenteeism. Economists have speculated about

the impact of increased mortality rates on the lifetime costs of obesity; some have

proposed that earlier mortality may offset increased obesity-related costs.

This dissertation develops a model of the lifetime, external costs of obesity in the United

States in two phases. Phase One is a meta-analysis of the obesity-related costing

literature, which informs cost categories and estimates in the subsequent phase. Phase

Two is the development of a Markov model using simulation software, which calculates

the lifetime, external costs of a hypothetical, 1000-person, obese cohort in comparison to

one of normal weight.

Results from the model developed here suggest that lifetime, external costs of obese

adults are on average $54,579 ($2007) greater per person than those of normal weight.

Using this estimate, which is likely conservative, if all 9 million obese children in the United States become obese adults, it would represent a lifetime, external cost of almost $500 billion.

The findings of the analysis presented here suggest that there are substantial financial externalities associated with obesity. Other obesity-related market failures may include information failure and imperfect rationality. Results from the present study suggest that government intervention to reduce obesity rates is warranted.

Table of Contents

Glossary of Terms

Adiposity

Body fatness. Adipose tissue in the body stores energy in the form of fat.

Body Mass Index / Obesity in Adults

Body Mass Index (BMI) is a standard by which weight status is determined. It is derived

from height and weight measurements, and may be calculated by dividing kilograms by

meters squared (kg/m^2). Using pounds and inches, the formula is: (weight in pounds /

height in inches)^2 x 703. The table below provides the classification of weight status by

BMI, which has been "adopted by the Expert Panel on the Identification, Evaluation, and

Treatment of Obesity in Adults and endorsed by leading organizations of health

professionals" (National Institutes of Health [NIH], 1998, p. 1). Please note that the term

"morbid obesity" is used synonymously throughout this dissertation with the term

"extreme obesity" and "obesity class III".

BMI Classification

	Obesity Class	**BMI (kg/m^2)**
Underweight		< 18.5
Normal		18.5-24.9
Overweight		25.0-29.9
Obesity	I	30.0-34.9
	II	35.0-39.9
Extreme Obesity	III	≥ 40

Source: National Institutes of Health (NIH), 1998

BMI is used widely as a measure of adiposity (NIH, 2004). Under some circumstances

however, BMI may not be an accurate measure of overweight or obesity. Individuals with

increased muscle mass relative to their height—such as athletes— may be described

incorrectly as overweight or obese. However, the number of individuals in the general

US population who fall into this category is likely small. A recent study that used objective measures of physical activity found that fewer than 5% of US adults are active 30 minutes per day (Troiano et al., 2008). Researchers such as Steven Blair have examined the effect of physical activity independent of bodyweight on health outcomes and argue that BMI alone is insufficient as a measure for adverse health outcomes (Blair, 2003; Lee, Jackson, & Blair, 1998). Nevertheless, BMI is used widely and is a broadly accepted measure of body fatness in research (NIH, 1998). Therefore, BMI is used as a measure of adiposity in the study presented here.

Cohort

Cohort is an epidemiologic term[1] used to describe a group of people followed over time for research purposes.

Incidence

Incidence is an epidemiologic term used to denote new cases of an illness or condition.

Morbidity

Morbidity is a general term referring to illness, health condition or event.

Mortality

Mortality is often used in epidemiology to denote the mortality rate, or number of deaths in a population.

---

[1] Explanations for epidemiologic terms in the glossary have been adapted from Aschengrau and Seage, 2003.

Odds Ratio and Relative Risk

Odds Ratio and *Relative Risk* are similar terms in epidemiology used to describe the risk

of an illness or condition relative to another population. However, their definitions differ

statistically. An *Odds Ratio* is used when researchers do not know the total population

from which the cases derive. The term *Relative Risk* is used when the total population of

the cases is known.

Overweight and Obesity in Children

Defining obesity in children is less straightforward than in adults. Firstly, there are

differences in terminology used in studies; some researchers do not use the term

"obesity" at all when describing children, and instead use "overweight" (Flegal, Tabak, &

Ogden, 2006). Secondly, the measurement of excess adiposity is different in children

compared to adults. As children are still growing and normal BMI levels vary across

different age groups, measures of childhood BMI are ranked relative to children at the

same age of a similar height and weight. The Centers for Disease Control and Prevention

created weight for height charts in children based on data from nationally representative

surveys (Kuczmarski et al., 2002). The 85th and 95th percentiles are generally used to

correspond to adult levels of overweight and obesity, respectively (Flegal et al., 2006).

In this dissertation, children whose BMI is greater than the 85th, but less than the 95th

percentile are referred to as "overweight", and children at the 95th percentile or greater

are referred to as "obese".

Prevalence

Prevalence is an epidemiologic term used to denote the number of existing cases of an

illness or condition

xxii

Chapter One: Policy Problem

Introduction

This dissertation examines obesity in the context of market failure. Obesity prevalence in the United States has risen dramatically in the last several decades. Over two thirds of the country is overweight and one third is considered obese, with racial/ethnic minorities at increased risk for both overweight and obesity. These trends show few signs of abating. Obesity is a risk factor for a wide range of chronic diseases, debilitating conditions, and mental health issues, including heart disease, diabetes, cancer, stroke, osteoarthritis, and depression. However, in addition to the human costs, there are significant economic ramifications to the sequelae of obesity. These include for example, increased healthcare costs, and higher rates of disability and absenteeism.

Economists have debated whether increased obesity prevalence constitutes an example of market failure and therefore justifies government intervention. Relatively few studies have calculated lifetime costs of obesity, and none has estimated its lifetime, external costs at the individual level. External costs are those that are not borne by the individual, but by other actors, such as insurance companies, employers, or by society. The research question examined in this dissertation is: *What are the lifetime, external costs of a 1000-person obese cohort in the United States, in comparison to one of normal weight?*

This dissertation develops a model of the lifetime external costs of obesity. It draws (1) conceptually from the studies by Manning, Keeler, Newhouse, Sloss, and Wasserman (1989; 1991) and Keeler, Manning, Newhouse, Sloss, and Wasserman (1989) on the lifetime, external costs of smoking, excessive alcohol consumption and lack of physical activity, and (2) methodologically from a more recent study by Tucker, Palmer, Valentine, Roze, and Ray (2006), which calculated lifetime costs of healthcare and quality of life related to obesity. The results of this dissertation may contribute to the economic literature on obesity and market failure and inform the debate regarding government intervention in reducing obesity rates.

This chapter provides background information on the issue of increased obesity prevalence in the United States and proceeds as follows: First, trend and socio-demographic information on obesity is provided. Second, information on the health and other economic effects of obesity is discussed. Third, correlates and causal influences on the rise of obesity in the United States are reviewed. The chapter concludes with an overview of the dissertation, and provides further information on the research question's significance and methodology.

Obesity Trends

Adults in the United States

Prevalence of overweight and obesity in the United States has risen significantly over the last fifty years, particularly since the mid-1970s. At the time of the first national health survey conducted by the National Center for Health Statistics (NCHS) in 1960-1962, obesity prevalence amongst US adults was 13.3%. In 2003-2004, the figure had risen to

33.9%. Combined prevalence of overweight and obesity rose from 44.8% to 67.1% in

the same period. Figure 1.1 shows this increase of overweight and obesity in adults in the

United States aged 20-74 (age-adjusted), in the non-institutionalized population.

Figure 1.1: US Trends in Prevalence of Overweight and Obesity in Adults

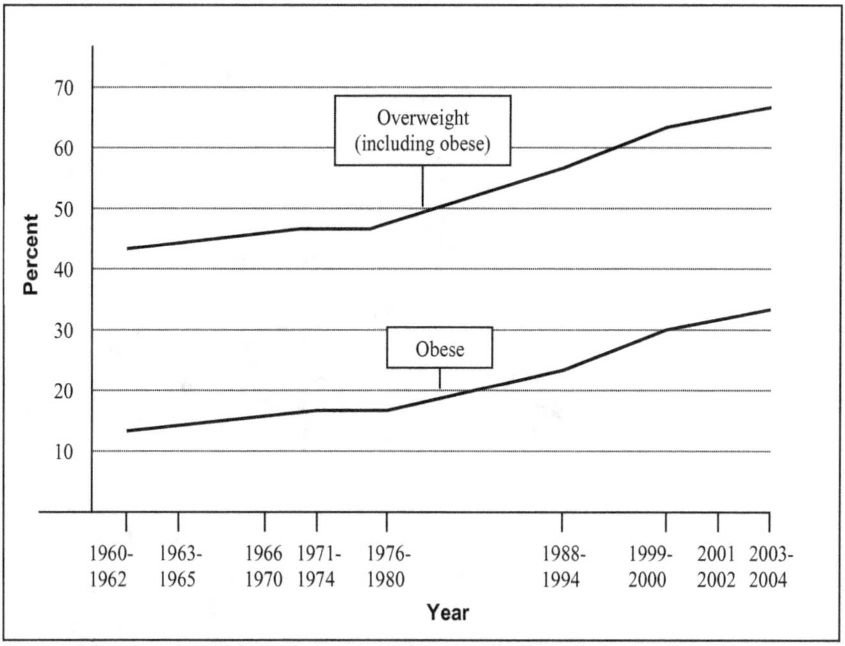

Source: Flegal et al., 2000; Ogden et al., 2002; NCHS 2006; Ogden et al., 2006

Figure 1.2 also displays obesity trend information for US adults, using state-by-state

information in the last 20 years. This data is drawn from the annual Behavioral Risk

Factor Surveillance System (BRFSS) survey, conducted by the Centers for Disease

Control and Prevention (CDC).

Figure 1.2: Obesity of US Adults by State: 1988, 1998, 2007

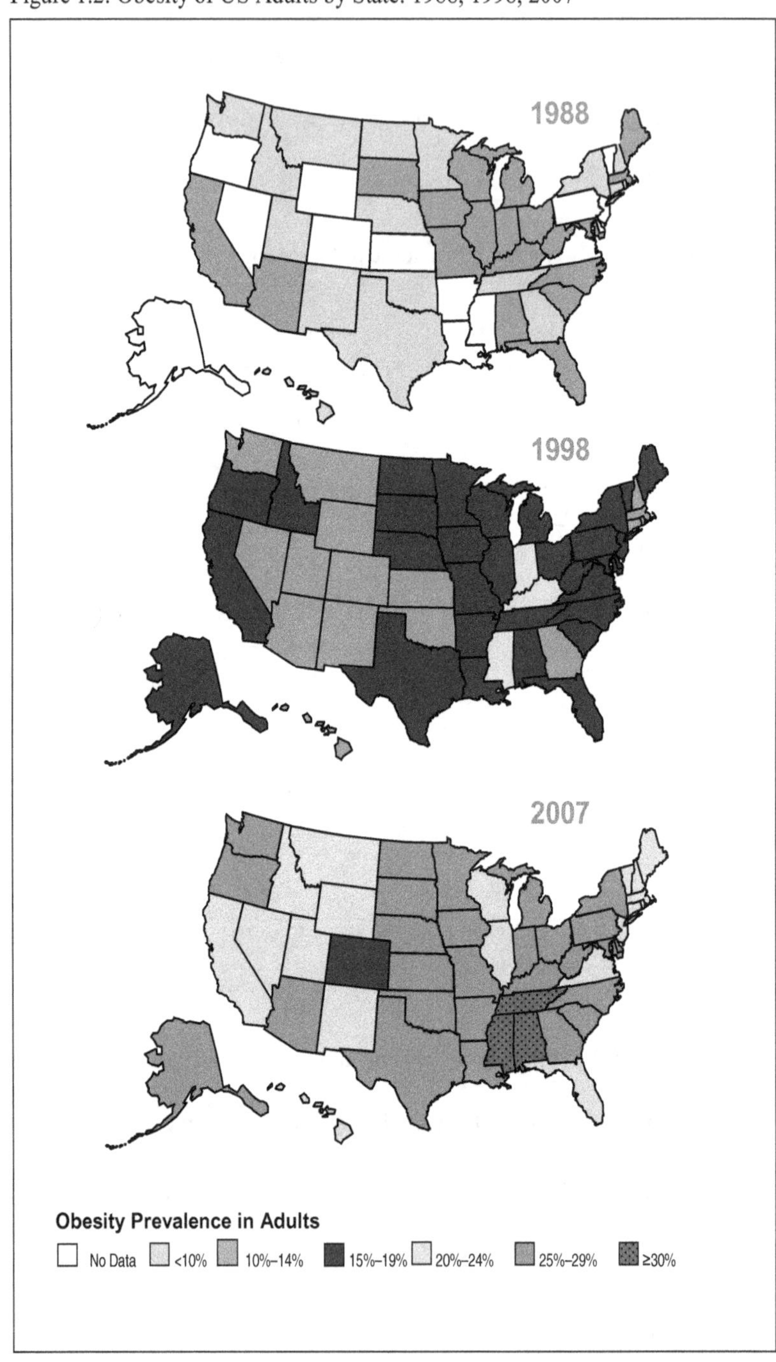

Source: Centers for Disease Control and Prevention (CDC), 2008

Children and Adolescents in the United States

Obesity trends in children and adolescents in the United States show a similar increase to

that in adults in the same period, as seen in Figure 1.3. Since the 1970s, obesity

prevalence has doubled in children, and tripled in adolescents. A report from the Institute

of Medicine (IOM) in 2005 stated that approximately nine million children in the United

States over the age of six were classified as overweight (Koplan, Liverman & Kraak,

2005).

Figure 1.3: US Trends in Prevalence of Obesity in Children

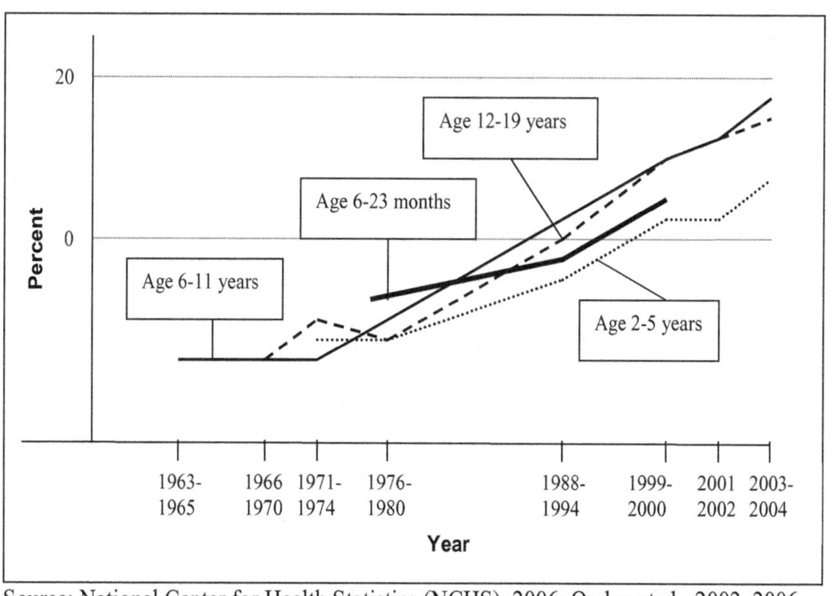

Source: National Center for Health Statistics (NCHS), 2006; Ogden et al., 2002, 2006

Obesity and the International Experience

The United States has the highest levels of overweight and obesity among developed

countries (World Health Organization [WHO], 2005), however, rising obesity levels is an

issue that affects developed and developing countries alike (Friedrich, 2002; James,

2004; WHO, 2005, 2006). The World Health Organization (WHO) reports that in 2005, there were 400 million obese adults (over the age of 15) worldwide, and 1.6 billion adults

who were overweight. Further, they predict that by 2015, the numbers will rise to 700

million and 2.3 billion, respectively (WHO, 2006). Obesity levels appear to be rising

most rapidly in those countries transitioning to a market economy (IARC, 2002). Figure

1.4 displays information on actual and projected figures for obesity rates in countries at

multiple income levels.

Figure 1.4: World Obesity (BMI ≥ 30) Levels in 2002 and Projected Figures for 2010 in
Persons ≥15 years

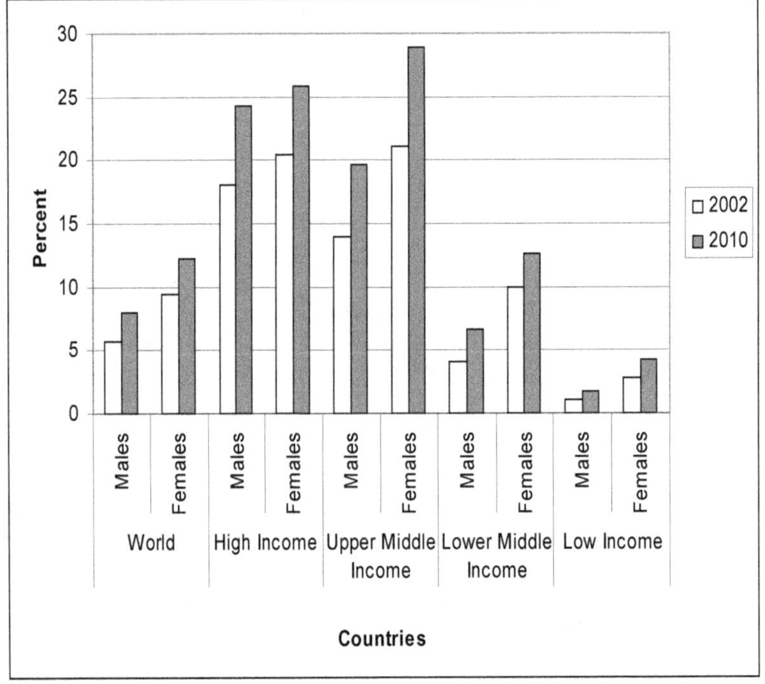

Source: Yach, Stuckler, & Brownell, 2006

In summary, it is clear that obesity rates in the United States have risen in the last 50

years, particularly over the last several decades. This change has occurred both in adults

and in children. Further, this rise in obesity prevalence has been a global trend. Having reviewed obesity trends, the following section examines the socio-demographics of obesity in the United States.

Socio-Demographics of Obesity

Race/Ethnicity: Adults

Average rates of overweight, obesity, and extreme (often termed "morbid") obesity in the 2003-2004 National Health and Nutrition Examination Survey (NHANES) were 66.3%, 32.2% and 4.8% respectively, however, obesity rates differ between racial and ethnic groups, and by socioeconomic status (SES) (Ogden et al., 2006). Rates of obesity and overweight are higher for Mexican-Americans and non-Hispanic blacks, in comparison to non-Hispanic whites. Non-Hispanic black women show the highest rates of obesity and in 2003-2004, 81.6% were overweight, 53.9% were obese, and 14.7% were extremely obese (Ogden et al. 2006), as seen in Figure 1.5.

Figure 1.5: Overweight, Obesity and Extreme Obesity Prevalence in the United States by Race/Ethnicity, 2003-2004

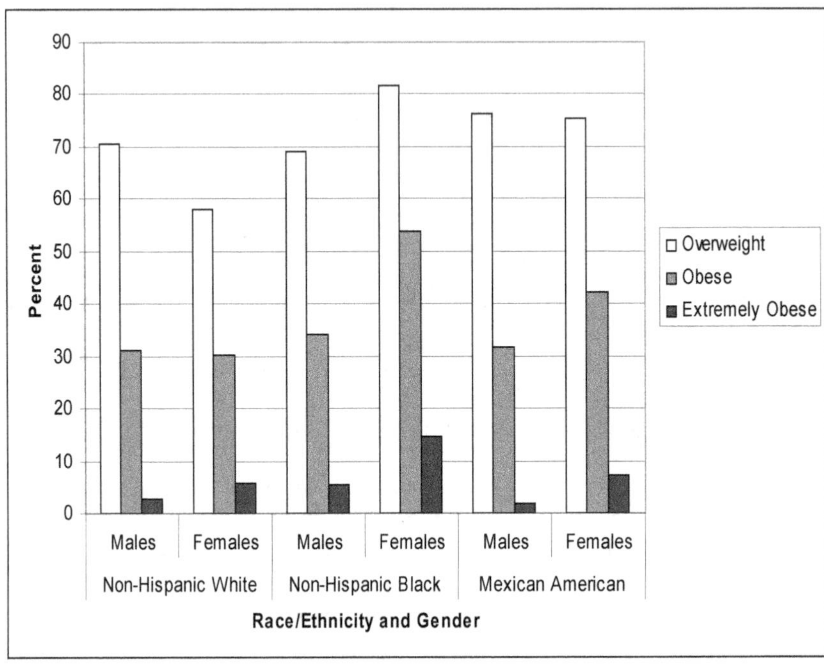

Source: (Ogden et al., 2006)

Race/Ethnicity: Children

The percentage of children who are overweight or obese also differs by race and

ethnicity, as seen in Figure 1.6. Mexican American boys and non-Hispanic black girls

show particularly high levels of obesity overall, and selected age groups within these

populations show yet higher levels. For example, 45.6% of non-Hispanic black girls

aged 6-11 and 47.9% of Mexican American boys aged 6-11 years are overweight or

obese (Ogden et al., 2006).

Figure 1.6: Obesity in US Children Aged 2-19 by Race/Ethnicity 2003-2004

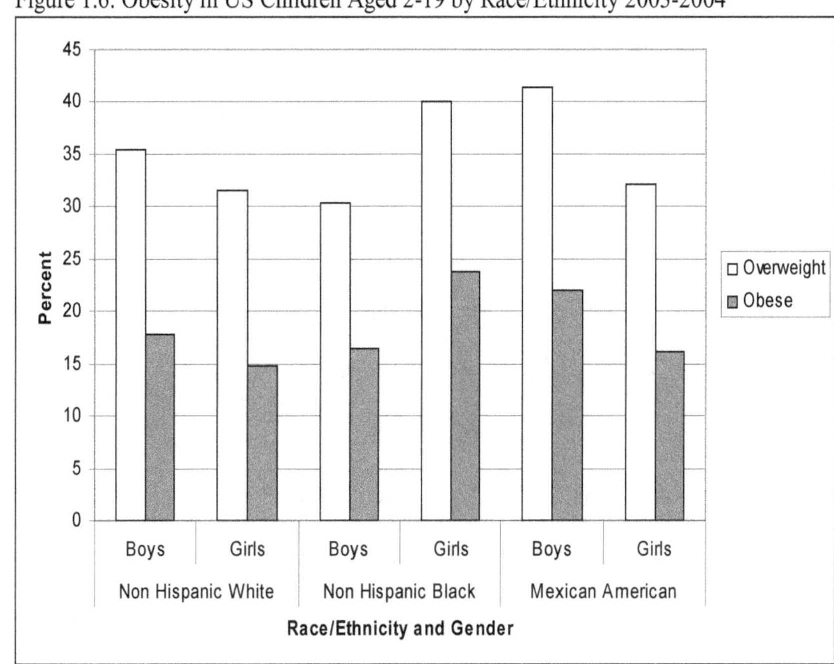

Source: (Ogden, 2006)

Native Americans are not included in the figures 1.5 or 1.6 as the NHANES survey, from which the figures derive, does not have a large enough sample of Native Americans to generate nationally representative data. However, while there is variation across tribes and communities, prevalence of overweight and obesity in Native American communities is generally higher than rates for the general US population, both in children and adults (Story et al., 2003).

Socioeconomic Status

Socioeconomic status (SES), which is usually measured by education level and income, is not consistently related to overweight and obesity prevalence. In adults, SES is inversely associated with obesity, however, this effect is mostly due to the association in women (Gortmaker, Must, Perrin, Sobol, & Dietz, 1993; DHHS 2001; Loucks et al., 2006; Stunkard, 1993). A 2005 report by the United States Department of Agriculture's (USDA) Economic Research Service (ERS) found that food stamp recipients were more likely to be obese than those with higher incomes, but this difference was due to the increased risk in women only (Lin, 2005). Gibson also found that participation in the food stamp program (now known as the Supplemental Nutrition Assistance Program, or SNAP) was positively correlated with obesity in women, but not in men (Gibson, 2003).

The relationship between income and obesity is more complex with children and teens. For example, Troiano and Flegal (1998) found in a study of National Health Examination Survey (NHES) and NHANES I, II and III data that obesity in children did not vary significantly with regard to income or education. However, other studies do show some variation. According to Kumanyika and Grier (2006), low-income children generally are at increased risk of obesity, and differences exist between different racial and ethnic groups. Lin (2002) also found that children of food stamp program recipients were more likely to be overweight. Miech et al. (2006) reported that older teens (15-17 years) in families below the poverty line were at increased risk of obesity compared to those above, but that this was not the case for mid-age teens (12-14 years). A study using data from the National Longitudinal Study of Adolescent Health found that an inverse relationship existed between SES-levels in white female adolescents and overweight, but not in white males, or other ethnic and racial groups (Gordon-Larsen, Adair & Popkin, 2003). Further, the study found that in African-American girls, SES levels were *positively* associated with increased levels of overweight. These results are similar to other studies

(Kimm, Obarzarnek & Barnek, 1996; Must, Gortmaker & Dietz, 1994)

The socio-demographics of obesity are therefore complex. Racial and ethnic minorities

clearly have higher rates of obesity, both in children and in adults. In contrast, the

relationship between bodyweight and other factors such as gender and income is less

straightforward. The next section reviews the health and economic consequences of

overweight and obesity.

Health and Economic Consequences of Obesity

Having reviewed the trends and socio-demographics related to obesity, this section

provides information on the health and economic effect of obesity. Both mortality and

morbidity information are reviewed in the following sections. Understanding these

health ramifications is important, given the potential impact to the nation's healthcare

system. The economic ramifications of rising obesity rates are only briefly discussed, as

these are covered in detail in subsequent chapters of this dissertation.

Mortality

Experts debate the precise effects of overweight and obesity on mortality. Estimates of

obesity's impact on annual US mortality range from 112,000 deaths (Flegal, Graubard,

Williamson & Gail, 2005) to 365,000 (Mokdad, Marks, Stroup, & Gerberding, 2005). In

1993, a study concluded that 14% of deaths in the US were related to poor diet and

inactivity (McGinnis & Foege, 1993). Calle, Thun, Petrelli, Rodriguez, & Heath (1999) found a U shaped relationship between BMI and mortality in a cohort study of over a million adults, however, another study found a J shaped relationship (Manson et al., 1995). The variation of these estimates may be due to the representativeness of a cohort relative to the general population, statistical methods and measures used in studies, in addition to advances in disease treatment.

Despite differences in describing the precise nature of the relationship and overall mortality rates, experts agree that BMI is correlated with an increased risk of mortality, particularly at high levels (Calle et al., 1999; Manson et al., 1995; NIH, 1998; National Task Force on the Prevention and Treatment of Obesity [NTFPTO], 2000). For example, Fontaine, Redden, Wang, Westfall and Allison (2003) have calculated that 20-year old white men with BMI levels of 30, 35, 40 and 45 would lose 1, 2, 6 and 13 years of life, respectively. Other researchers have even suggested that increased levels of obesity levels may lead to an overall decline in life expectancy in the United States in the 21st century (Olshansky et al., 2005).

Morbidity

A wide range of health issues is associated with overweight and obesity. According to Sturm, (2004), the impact of obesity on chronic health issues is similar to the effects of aging 20 years. The health conditions associated with overweight and obesity may be broken into the following categories: chronic diseases, debilitating conditions and psychosocial issues (Kumanyika, Jeffery, Morabia, Ritenbaugh, & Antipatis, 2002).

Table 1.1 shows the morbidity associated with obesity, and the sections below provide

information on several of these diseases and conditions, and their linkages to obesity.

Table 1.1 Selected Health Conditions Associated with Overweight and Obesity

Chronic Diseases	Type 2 diabetes
	Coronary heart disease
	Cancer
	Stroke
	Hypertension
	Osteoarthritis
	Gallbladder and liver disease
Debilitating Conditions	Respiratory issues, e.g., sleep apnea, asthma
	Reproductive issues, e.g., infertility, complications in pregnancy
Psychosocial Issues	Clinical depression
	Reduced self-esteem
	Social stigma

Source: (Kopelman, 2007; Kumayika et al., 2002; Must et al., 1999; NTFPTO, 2000; Pi-Sunyer, 2002)

Diabetes

Diabetes is a cluster of diseases marked by increased blood glucose levels (National

Institute for Digestive and Diabetes and Kidney Diseases [NIDDK], 2005). If not

managed appropriately, diabetes may increase the risk of heart disease and stroke, high

blood pressure, blindness, kidney disease, amputations, periodontal disease, and

premature death (NIDDK, 2005). In 2005, of the population in the US aged 20 and older,

20.6 million had diabetes (9.6% of the population ≥20 years); of the population aged 60

and older, 10.3 million had diabetes (20.9% of the population ≥60 years) (NIDDK,

2005). The three most common forms of diabetes include type 1, type 2 and gestational

diabetes (NIDDK, 2005). Type 1 is an autoimmune disorder where the body in incapable

of creating insulin and presents in childhood and accounts for 5-10% of cases; type 2 diabetes (also known as 'adult onset diabetes') represents 90-95% of diabetes cases; gestational diabetes affects some women during pregnancy only (NIDDK, 2005). Type 2 and gestational diabetes are the forms of diabetes most closely associated with obesity.

There is a strong, curvilinear relationship between diabetes type 2 and obesity (Colditz, Willett, Rotnitzky, & Manson, 1995; Field et al., 2001; Li, Bowerman, & Heber, 2005; Must et al., 1999). This association is seen even at BMI levels considered in the normal range. For example, a report from a large cohort study found that in comparison to a woman whose BMI was less than 22, the risk of developing diabetes was five times greater at a BMI of 24-24.9, 15.8 times greater at BMIs of 27-28.9 and rose to 93 times greater at BMIs of 35 and above (Colditz et al., 1995).

Researchers have estimated that 80-90% of type 2 diabetes cases may be attributed to the combination of inactivity and overweight/obesity (Kumanyika et al., 2002; Stein & Colditz, 2004). Studies show that even modest weight loss reduces one's risk of developing diabetes (Li et al., 2005). Trends of population-level prevalence of diabetes type 2 appear ominous. Research suggests that if obesity rates remain at current levels, a boy born in 2000 has a 30% chance of developing the disease, a girl: almost 40% (Narayan, Boyle, Thompson, Sorensen & Williamson, 2003). Diabetes type 2 is also appearing at earlier stages; incidence in children and teens has increased significantly in the US and internationally in recent years (Pinhas-Hamel & Zeitler, 2005).

Cancer

In 2004, cancer was the second most common disease-related cause of death United States, responsible for over 23% of deaths, and according to analysis of 2002-2004 data, the lifetime risk of dying from cancer was almost 41% (Ries et al., 2007). Research suggests there is a causal linkage between overweight/obesity and cancer-related morbidity and mortality. A report by the International Agency for Research on Cancer (IARC) determined that there was sufficient evidence to establish a causal link between obesity and cancers of the colon, breast (postmenopausal), endometrium, kidney and esophagus (International Agency for Research on Cancer [IARC], 2002). Further, the report found that approximately 9% of post-menopausal breast cancer, 37% esophageal cancer, 25% of kidney cancer and 39% of endometrial cancer was attributable to increased BMI levels (IARC, 2002). A large prospective cohort study of adults in the United States found that overweight and obesity was linked to increased mortality by cancers of the: esophagus, colon, rectum, liver, gallbladder, pancreas, kidney, stomach, prostate, breast, uterus, cervix, ovary, as well as non-Hodgkins lymphoma and multiple myeloma (Calle, Rodriguez, Walker-Thurmond, & Thun, 2003). For non-smokers, obesity may be the leading avoidable cause of cancer, and overall may account for 14% of deaths due to cancer in men, and 20% in women (Calle & Thun, 2004).

Coronary Heart Disease

Coronary Heart Disease (CHD) is the result of narrowed arteries in the heart due to deposits of fat and/or cholesterol; when constricted, these narrowed passages may result in angina or even heart attack (National Heart, Lung, and Blood Institute [NHLBI], nd).

CHD is the leading cause of death in the United States (Ries et al., 2007), and is responsible for over 650,000 deaths annually (Minino, Heron, & Smith, 2006), and is highly correlated with levels of obesity (Minino et al., Must et al., 1999; Pi-Sunyer, 2002; Stein & Colditz, 2004). Analysis from the Nurses' Health Study—a large and long-running cohort study of nurses currently led by researchers at the Harvard School of Public Health (Nurses Health Study [NHS], 2008)—found that in comparison to a woman whose BMI was under 22, mortality from cardiovascular disease was 3.1, 4.6 and 5.8 times greater for women whose BMI was 27-28.9, 29-31.9, and ≥32, respectively (Manson et al., 1995).

Hypertension

Hypertension, or high blood pressure, is defined as a blood pressure reading of 140/90 mmHg or higher (NHLBI, 2006). Hypertension increases the risk of CHD, stroke, kidney disease, and blindness. Hypertension affects more that 25% of the US population (National Center for Health Statistics [NCHS], 2006), and is linearly related to overweight and obesity. According to one study, men who are overweight, obese, and extremely obese are 2.4, 3.8 and 4.2 times more likely to develop hypertension than their leaner peers over a ten year period (Field et al., 2001).

Stroke

Stroke is the third leading cause of death in the United States, and a leading cause of long-term disability (Ries et al., 2007; Stein & Colditz, 2004). Increased BMI also may increase one's risk of ischemic, but not hemorrhagic stroke[2] (NTFPTO, 2000). Research

from the Nurses Health Study found that women whose BMI levels were ≥ 27 were

roughly twice as likely to develop ischemic stroke than women whose BMI levels were

less than 21 (Rexrode, et al., 1997). The ten-year risk of developing stroke was two and a

half times greater for severely obese men than those men whose BMI levels were 18.5-

21.9 (Field et al., 2001).

Psychosocial Issues

Obesity in adults is associated with increased risk for depression, however, research

suggests that effects may be stronger in women at lower grades of obesity than in men

(de Wit, van Straten, van herten, Pennix & Cuipers, 2009; Fabricatore & Wadden, 2006;

Zhao et al., 2009). In addition, psychosocial issues resulting from obesity in childhood

may be significant (Dietz, 1998; Ebbeling, Pawlak, & Ludwig, 2002). According to

Schwimmer, Burwinkle, & Varni (2003), obese children reported health-related quality

of life below that of healthy children. Severely obese children and teens reported quality

of life levels similar to that of pediatric cancer patients (Schwimmer et al., 2003). In

adults, obesity is linked at the same or higher rate to decreased quality of life than recent

heavy alcohol consumption, smoking or poverty (Sturm & Wells, 2001).

Graphical Representations of Morbidity

This section provides illustrations of selected information from the previous sub-sections.

Five conditions associated with obesity include gallstones, hypertension, colon cancer,

---

[2] Ischemic stroke involves blockages to the blood vessels in the brain, while hemorrhagic stroke results in blood vessel rupture.

heart disease and type 2 diabetes. Figures 1.7 and 1.8 show the ten-year risks of

developing the first four of these conditions by BMI, according to the results from two

large cohort studies. For example, the odds of a man with a BMI ≥35 developing

hypertension over a ten-year period are more than four times greater than a man whose

BMI is 18.5-21.9.

Figure 1.7: Ten Year Risk of Developing Obesity-Related Diseases: Men

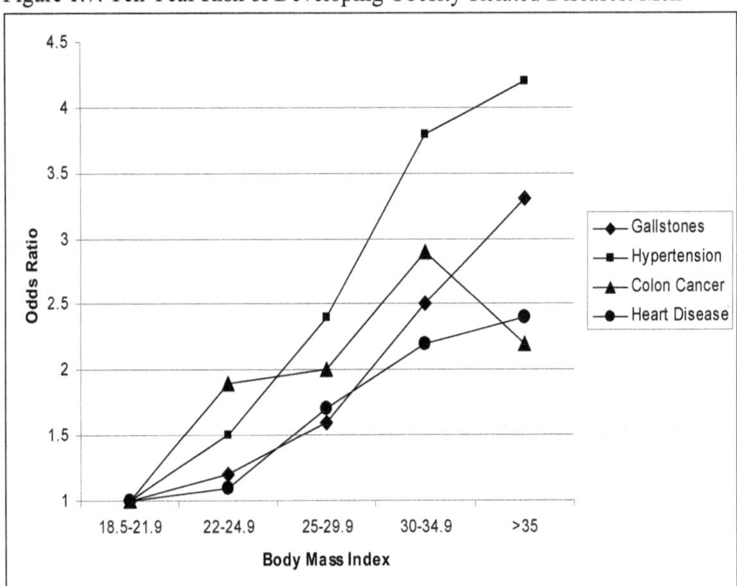

Source: Must et al., 1999

Figure 1.8: Ten Year Risk of Developing Obesity-Related Diseases: Women

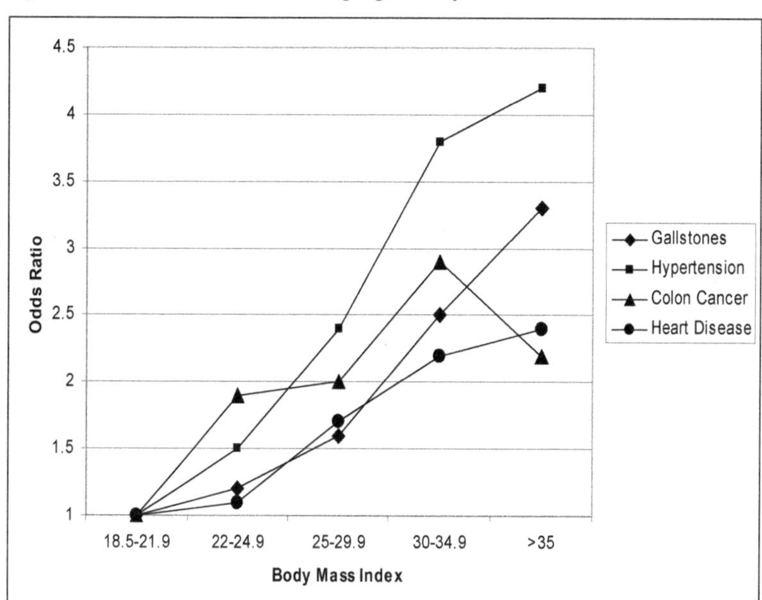

Source: Must et al., 1999

However, the risks associated with type 2 diabetes dwarfs that of the health conditions

shown in Figures 1.7 and 1.8. Figures 1.9 and 1.10 show the risks associated with

gallstones, hypertension, colon cancer and heart disease in men and women—the same

information displayed in Figures 1.7 and 1.8—when diabetes type 2 is included in the

chart.

Figure 1.9: Ten Year Risk of Developing Obesity-Related Diseases: Men; Includes
Diabetes Type 2

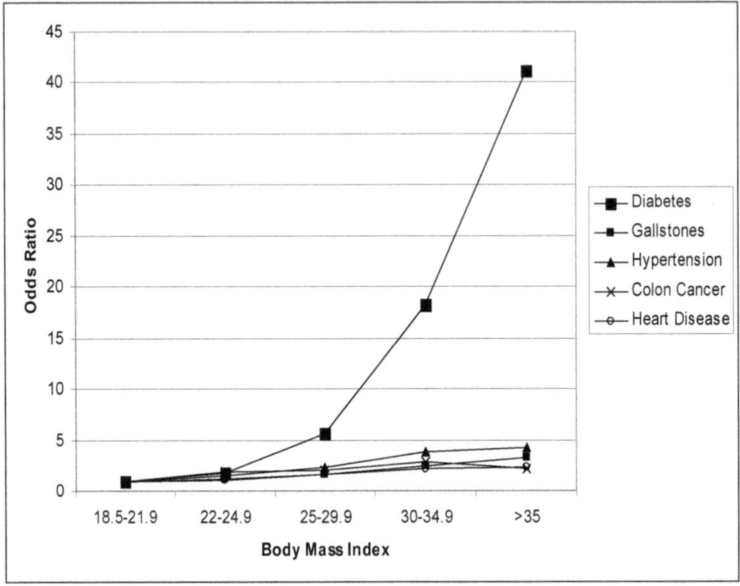

Source: Must et al, 1999

Figure 1.10: Ten Year Risk of Developing Obesity-Related Diseases: Women; Includes
Diabetes Type 2

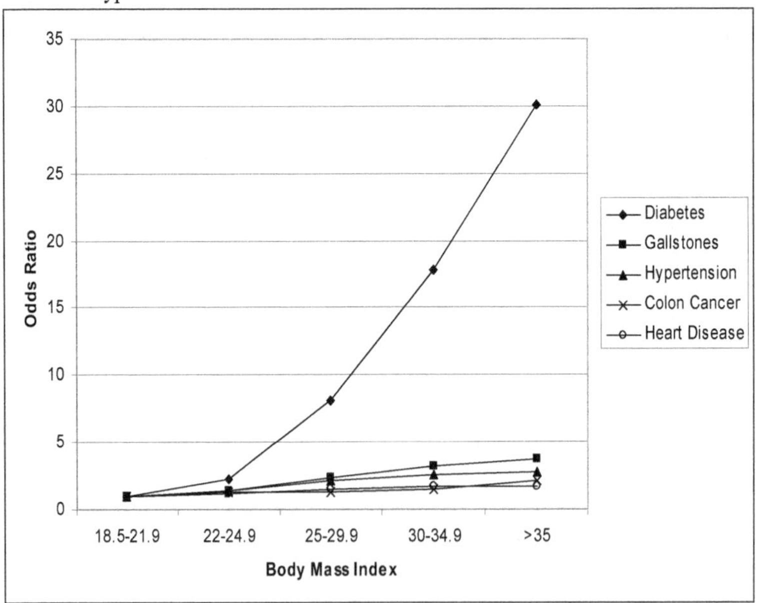

Source: Must et al., 1999

Health Implications of Obesity in Children

Obesity in childhood is a strong predictor of obesity in adulthood (Steinberger, Moran, Hong, Jacobs, & Sinaiko, 2001). In addition, it appears that the likelihood an obese child will become an obese adult increases with his or her age. An obese four-year old has a 20% chance of become obese in adulthood, an obese adolescent: 80% (Guo & Chumlea, 1999; Krebs, 2003). Two recent studies suggest that obesity in childhood increases the likelihood of coronary heart disease in adulthood (Baker, Olsem, & Sorenson, 2007; Bibbins-Domingo, Coxson, Pletcher, Lightwood, & Goldman, 2007), and other research suggests that obesity in early adulthood may significantly lower life expectancy (Fontaine, Redden, Wang, Westfall, & Allison, 2003).

Economic Consequences of Obesity

In addition to health-related consequences, the economic ramifications of obesity appear to be substantial. The economic impact of obesity is the subject of this dissertation and the following chapters will discuss the obesity-related costs in detail. However, to provide context, some information on the economic impact of obesity is provided here.

Obesity appears to account for a sizeable proportion of US healthcare spending, and to be an important contributor to rising healthcare costs. Finkelstein, Fiebelkorn, and Wang (2003) estimated that in 1998, obesity-related healthcare costs represented 9.1% of healthcare spending in the US ($78.5 billion in $1998; $105.9 billion in $2008), half of which is financed by Medicare and Medicaid. Thorpe, Florence, Howard, and Joski (2004) estimated that 27% of the rise in healthcare spending in the US between 1987 and

2001 was due to obesity, and according to Sturm (2002), obesity outranks smoking and excess alcohol use in its impact to healthcare costs. In addition, obesity appears to increase costs associated with absenteeism, disability and reduced productivity (Finkelstein, Fiebelkorn, & Wang 2005).

The impact of obesity on healthcare costs is not limited to the United States, although the percentage impact of obesity on healthcare spending appears lower in other countries. Researchers have estimated obesity-related costs for many other countries, including Switzerland (Schmid, Schneider, Golay, & Keller, 2005), Canada (Birmingham, Muller, Palepu, Spinelli, & Anis, 1999; Katzmarzyk & Janssen, 2004), Japan (Kuriyama, 2006), the United Kingdom (Allender & Rayner, 2007), Germany (Sander & Burgemann, 2003), Australia (Segal, Carter, & Zimmet, 1994), the Netherlands (Seidell, 1995), and France (Lévy, 1995). Costs associated with obesity in these countries range from 2% of total healthcare expenditure in France (E. Lévy, P. Lévy, Le Pen, & Basdevant, 1995) to 4% in the Netherlands (Seidell, 1995).

In summary, although the specific nature of the relationship between mortality and obesity is debated, the morbidities associated with obesity are serious, numerous, and well-supported by the data. There also appear to be significant direct and indirect economic costs of obesity, for example, health care costs and absenteeism. The next section examines why this rise in obesity prevalence has occurred on such a broad scale.

Correlates and Causal Influences of Obesity

This section investigates the correlates and causal influences implicated in the relatively recent increase in obesity prevalence. The causes of overweight and obesity appear to be simultaneously straightforward and complex. On one hand, weight gain results when energy intake exceeds expenditure, and evidence suggests that Americans have increased caloric intake over the last several decades and that there has not been a compensatory increase in energy expenditure over the same period. On the other hand, why these behavioral changes have occurred on such a broad scale is not known exactly, although many environmental variables are implicated.

The number of calories consumed appears to have exceeded calories burned for many Americans over the last several decades. According to the CDC, between 1971 and 2000, average daily caloric intake in the United States increased 168 calories for men (from 2450 to 2618), and 335 calories for women (from 1542 to1877) (CDC, 2004a). The IOM reports that average energy intake increased for children and adolescents between 80 and 230 calories over a similar period (IOM, 2002). Although physical activity levels and trends are more difficult to discern due to difficulties in measurement and existing surveillance systems (French, Story, & Jeffery, 2001), evidence suggests that physical activity levels have declined over the last several decades. According to the IOM Transportation Research Board: "Physical activity levels have declined sharply over the past half-century because of reduced physical demands of work, household management, and travel, together with increased sedentary uses of free time" (IOM, 2005). However, a report from the Surgeon General reported little change in leisure-time physical activity between 1985-1991 (US Department of Health and Human Services [DHHS], 1996).

CDC reported that from 1990-1998, leisure time physical activity increased very slightly

from 24.3% to 25.4%, and that there was a slight decrease in no leisure-time physical

activity between 1990 and 1998 from 30.7% to 28.7% (CDC, 2001).

The reason(s) for this large-scale change in energy-balance (dietary and physical activity)

behavior cannot be isolated to one or two specific changes. Rather, many small changes

are implicated. Behavioral scientists use social-ecological models to describe influences

on eating and physical activity patterns, and the resulting impact on energy balance. This

model, represented in Figure 1.11, is adapted from several examples (Glass & McAtee,

2006; Koplan et al., 2005; Kumanyika et al., 2002), and will be used as a framework in

the section below to discuss several correlates and causal influences suggested by the

literature on individual energy balance.

Figure 1.10: Social-Ecological Model of Energy Intake and Expenditure

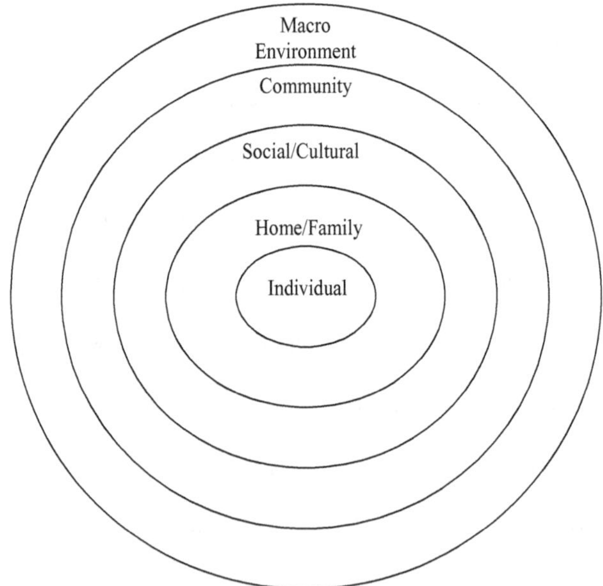

Individual Level

Genetics / Biology

Genetics and basic biology clearly influence individual adiposity. The ability for humans

to store excess energy as fat is critical to survival and reproduction and is likely to have

been an advantage to humans in evolutionary terms (Rosenbaum & Leibel, 1998). In

addition, humans appear to possess an innate preference for sweet and salty tastes (Birch

& Fisher, 1998). In a small percentage of cases, severe obesity may be the result of

genetic disorders (Farooqi & O'Rahilly, 2007). Absent a specific disorder however, there

also appears that heredity exerts a strong influence on susceptibility to overweight and

obesity (Garn et al., 1976; Stunkard, Harris, Pedersen, & McClearn, 1990; Whitaker,

Wright, Pepe, Seidel, & Dietz, 1997). Studies involving families and twins reared

together and apart, suggest that genes account for 45-75% in the variation of body weight

(Farooqi & O'Rahilly, 2007; Sorensen, Holst, & Stunkard, 1992; Stunkard et al., 1990). It

appears that there may be a general genetic susceptibility to overweight given the

appropriate environment (Rosenbaum & Leibel, 1998).

Pre-Natal Environment

The prenatal environment for a developing fetus also appears to influence obesity risk

later in life. A review article found that increased birth weight and maternal diabetes

were linked with increased body weight in adulthood, although the means by which this

occurred is not fully understood (Whitaker & Dietz, 1998).

Home/Family Level

Television Viewing

There is strong evidence that increased hours spent watching television is a causal influence on overweight and obesity (Dietz & Gortmaker, 1985; Gortmaker et al., 1996; Robinson, 1999). Less well established is the mechanism behind this link, but studies indicate that television viewing may: displace physical activity (Ebbeling et al., 2002); encourage unhealthy snacking (Francis, Lee & Birch, 2003); and/or promote consumption of high fat/high sugar foods through advertising (Boynton-Jarrett et al., 2003). A report from the Nurses' Health Study suggests that television-viewing was associated with increased obesity levels independent of exercise levels (Hu, Li, Coldtitz, Willett, & Manson, 2003).

Television ownership in the United States is high. Almost all (98%) of American homes have television sets, 88% have more than one, and 60% have three or more (Koplan et al., 2005; Roberts, Foehr, Rideout, & Brodie, 1999). Nielsen Media reports that in 2005, average daily television viewing in US households was at the highest level ever recorded at 8 hours and 11 minutes, an increase of almost 30% from 6 hours and 18 minutes in 1975 (Nielsen, 2005a, 2005b).

Breastfeeding

The percentage of infants who had ever been breastfed in the United States was close to the national goal of 75% at 71.4% in 2002, however, continuation of breastfeeding rates postpartum are well below target levels (Li, Darling, Maurice, Barker L, & Grummer-

Strawn, 2005). The lowest rates of breastfeeding in the US were found in non-Hispanic black infants and low-SES groups (Li et al., 2005; Ryan, Wenjun, & Acosta, 2002). Epidemiologic studies show that breast-feeding in infancy provides a small but measurable protective effect against obesity, although again, the mechanism by which this occurs are not fully understood (Anderson, Butcher, & Levine, 2003a; Koplan et al., 2005; Singhal & Lanigan, 2007; von Kries et al., 1999). One possibility is that breast-fed infants develop better satiety signals, whereas formula-fed babies may be encouraged to over-consume in order to finish a particular portion, thus disrupting development of this satiety mechanism (Koplan et al., 2005).

Maternal Employment

Maternal employment may influence overweight and obesity in children. The increase in women's participation in the labor force over the last four decades represents a major societal shift. From 1975 to 2005, the percentage of mothers with children younger than 18 in the paid workforce increased from 47 to 71%, peaking at 73% in 2005 (Bureau of Labor Statistics [BLS], 2006). Results of studies estimating the effects of maternal employment on childhood obesity have been mixed (Johnson, Smiciklas-Wright, Crouter, 1992). A study using data from the National Longitudinal Study of Youth (NLSY) that examined various subgroups of the population found a significant, causal relationship between maternal employment and overweight in children (Anderson et al., 2003a). The study found that among higher socio-economic groups, higher work intensity (increased number of hours a mother works per week over a child's life) was correlated with a higher likelihood of childhood obesity. The mechanism by which mothers' employment status may increase the likelihood of childhood obesity is not completely understood. However, it may be that in this particular group, increased maternal employment increases consumption of more energy-dense food that has been prepared outside the home (Anderson et al., 2003a).

Social/Cultural Level

Micro-Environment

Researchers at Cornell University have conducted a number of innovative experiments that suggest dietary behavior is influenced by unconscious, contextual effects of the "micro-environment". These micro-environmental, contextual effects include evidence of increased consumption, container size, and verbal cues of food/beverage origin. For example, researchers found in an experimental restaurant setting that participants who (unknowingly) ate from an automatically refilled soup bowl, consumed 73% more soup than their dinner partners who ate from regular soup bowls (Wansink, Painter, & North, 2005b). Further, diners with the refillable soup bowls were unaware of this increased consumption, and reported satiety levels similar to their dinner partners. Another experiment was conducted on moviegoers in Chicago, who received free, but stale popcorn, just after having eaten lunch (Wansink & Kim, 2005). Despite the absence of hunger and an unappetizing snack, moviegoers consumed 34% more popcorn from 240g containers than those who were provided 120g containers. Yet another study indicates that subtle contextual effects such as "sensory expectations" influence food intake. Restaurant-goers given a complimentary glass of wine ate 12% more food when told that the wine was from California, in comparison to when they were told their wine was from

North Dakota (Wansink, Painter, & North, 2007c).

Social Networks

Social networks may also influence obesity incidence (Christakis & Fowler, 2007). In an

analysis of a cohort of over 12,000 people from the Framingham Heart Study—a large

cohort study funded by NHLBI (Framingham Heart Study, 2008)—researchers found that

regardless of geography and blood relationship, one was more likely to gain or lose

weight if a friend or family member gained or lost weight (Christakis & Fowler, 2007).

Specifically, a person was more likely to become obese if a friend, sibling or spouse

became obese by 57%, 40% or 37%, respectively (Christakis & Fowler, 2007).

Portion Size

Portion size may be another contributing factor to general increased energy consumption.

Increased portion sizes may encourage consumers to choose these larger serving sizes as

they provide lower per unit costs (French et al., 2001; Young & Nestle, 2002). In the

1950s, 6.5oz bottles of Coca Cola represented 80% of sales, but today, a 20oz container

is the standard serving size (French et al., 2001). Young and Nestle (2002) found that

portion sizes, and therefore overall calories, in take-out, fast-food and family-style

restaurants increased substantially since the 1970s, and in many cases well exceeded

USDA and FDA portion sizes (Young & Nestle, 2002). In addition, Nielsen and Popkin

(2003) found that portion sizes and energy intakes for specific foods and beverages

(including: salty snacks, desserts, soft drinks, french fries, hamburgers, and pizza) had

increased significantly between 1977 and 1998 both in fast-food restaurants and in homes. These increased portions may be particularly significant given that research by

Wansink and Kim (2006) indicates that children and adults consume more when given, or

serve themselves, larger portions (Fisher, Liu, Birch, & Rolls, 2007; Wansink & Van

Ittersum, 2007; Wansink & Kim, 2006). It does not appear that people compensate for

this increased consumption by reducing intake in subsequent days (Rolls, Roe, &

Meengs, 2007).

Community Level

School Food Environment

Children in the United States are required to be in school seven hours per day, 180 days

per year, and the school food environment may have a significant impact on a child's

daily food consumption (DHHS, 2001; Kubik, Lytle, Hannan, Perry, Story M, 2003;

Wechsler, Devereaux, Davis, & Collins, 2000). Research suggests that 19-50% of a

child's daily caloric intake may be from the school cafeteria (Burghardt, Gordon,

Chapman, Gleason & Fraker, 1993).

Most school food service programs offer "competitive foods" for sale. Competitive foods

are all foods and beverages for sale in schools outside the federal school meal program,

and include food and beverages sold à la carte in school cafeterias, as well as in school

stores, vending machines and as fund-raisers (IOM 2004b; Story, Kaphingst & French,

2006). Most of these foods and beverages are high in fat and/or sugar and low in nutrients

(French, Story, Fulkerson, & Gerlach, 2003). Selling competitive food at school is

widespread, as shown in Figure 1.12.

Figure 1.11: Availability of Competitive Foods in Schools by Venue

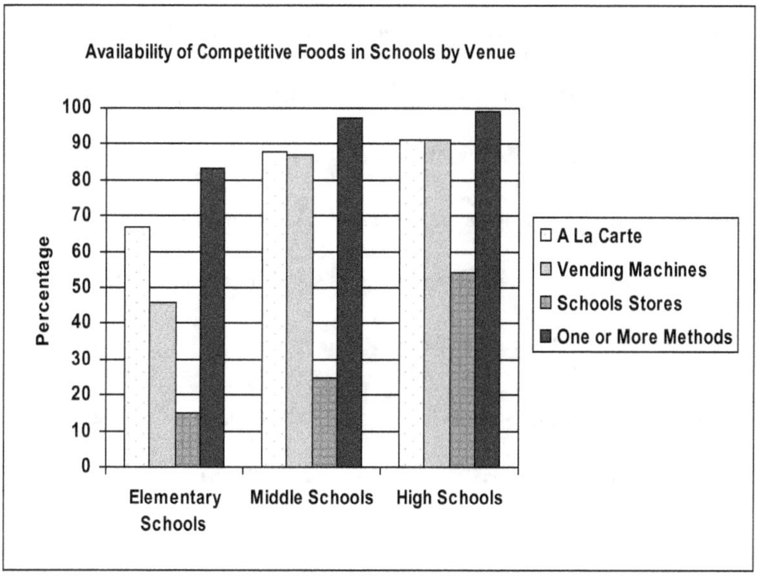

Source: Government Accountability Office [GAO], 2005

Research indicates that this widespread availability of high-calorie, nutrient-poor foods ("junk foods") negatively impact children and teen diets (McGinnis, Gootman, & Kraak, 2005). Energy-dense, nutrient-poor foods may displace more healthful choices. A recent study on the association between adolescents' dietary consumption and school vending machines and à la carte programs, found that availability of à la carte items was inversely associated with consumption of fruit and vegetables, and positively associated with total fat and saturated fat intake (Kubik et al., 2003). Another study by Anderson and Butcher (2006b) examined the effect of advertising and availability of junk food in schools and their findings suggested that a 10% increase in this exposure resulted in a 1% increase in adolescent BMI levels. However, these effects appeared to be limited to teens with at least one overweight parent, suggesting a possible gene-environment interaction (Anderson & Butcher, 2006b).

31

School-Related Physical Activity

In addition to energy intake, energy expenditure may also impact obesity rates. Many schools around the country have reduced physical education required of students (IOM, 2004b). A report from 2001 shows that slightly more than 50% of students in elementary school are required to participant in physical education, but this falls sharply in middle school and high school to 5.4% for grade 12, as shown in Figure 1.13 (Burgeson, Wechsler, Brener, Young, & Spain, 2001).

Figure 1.12: Percentage of Schools Requiring Physical Education by Grade, 2000

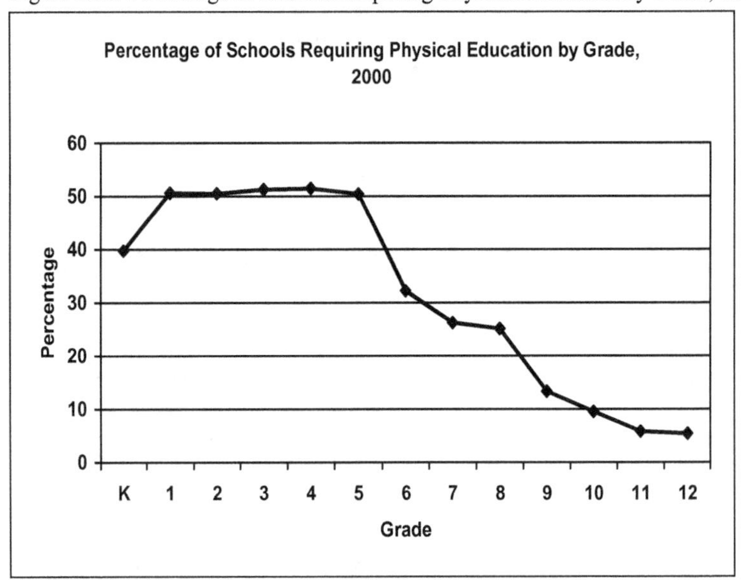

Source: Burgeson et al., 2001

According to data drawn from the 2003 Youth Risk Behavioral Surveillance (YRBS), over 33% of youth had not undertaken sufficient physical activity in the week before the survey, and 11% had not undertaken any physical activity (CDC, 2004b). Percentages in both categories were higher in African American and Hispanic youth than for whites, and higher in girls than boys (CDC, 2004b). This report notes that while enrollment in physical education remained relatively constant between 1991-2003, attendance dropped

markedly 1991-1995 from 41.6% to 25.4%, then remained relatively steady 1995-2003

(25.4% to 28.4%) (CDC, 2004b, 2004c). Cawley, Meyerhoefer, & Newhouse (2005)

examined the effect of state-based physical education regulations on student activity and

weight. Their results suggested that although regulations increased activity levels, this

did not affect BMI in children or teens, or their likelihood of being overweight.

A recent study of a nationally representative sample of children surveyed in 2002 found

that 22% walked or biked to school (Anderson & Butcher, 2006a). This contrasted

sharply with their parents, 70% of whom reported walking or biking to school 20-30

years earlier.

Built Environment Related to Physical Activity

The built environment—defined by the IOM as "land use patterns, the transportation

system, and design features that together provide opportunities for travel and physical

activity" (IOM, 2005, p. 2)—and its impact on energy balance and health, is a relatively

new area of inquiry (Frank, 2000). Studies in this area are largely cross-sectional rather

than longitudinal in design. Although correlations between physical activity levels and

the built environment are found (Saelens & Handy, 2008), the study designs often

prevent causal inference (IOM, 2005). However, it appears that changes in the built

environment may have served to decrease the "incidental" forms of physical activity

previously part of everyday life, thus contributing to the deficit in the energy balance

equation. Since the early 1950s, there has been a residential exodus from cities to the

suburbs, and thus from compact community design patterns to dispersed, where usually there are few sidewalks and driving is the most convenient form of transportation (Frank, 2000; IOM, 2005; Koplan et al., 2005). Although precise estimates of walking and biking for transportation are not available, it seems that there has been a shift from walking/biking to driving for transportation as a percentage of total trips, however the overall number of trips has increased (Sturm, 2004). As Eid, Overman, Puga, & Turner (2006) and Plantinga & Bernell (2005) note, future research on the effects of the built environment must take greater account of residents' self-selection into neighborhoods. Recent studies by Handy et al., (2006, 2008) attempt to control for residential self-selection, and find evidence that the built environment does influence physical activity by area residents.

Community Food Environment

Similar to the research on the impact of the built environment on activity levels, studies on the community food environment—defined here as food stores, restaurants, schools and worksites—and its potential impact on dietary behavior, is a relatively new research field. Study designs used in this research are generally cross-sectional, and therefore preclude inferring a causal connection between the community food environment, eating patterns and health/obesity. However, correlations have been found between neighborhood racial/ethnic profile, SES, and food access, price and quality. For example, studies have found associations between the density of fast-food restaurants and African American and/or low-income populations (Lewis et al., 2005; Block, Scribner, & DeSalvo, 2004). Evidence exists that some communities in the United States may have reduced access to nutritious and affordable food, that is, they may be "food deserts".

Studies that support the existence of food deserts in the US include: Chung and Myers, 1999; Morland, Wing, Diez-Roux & Poole 2002; Sloane et al., 2003; Horowitz Colson, Hebert and Lancaster, 2004; Block and Kouba, 2006; Zenk et al, 2005; Hendricksen, Smith and Eikenberry, 2006; Hosler, Varadarajulu, Ronsani, Frederick and Fisher, 2006; Jetter and Cassady, 2006; Moore and Diez-Roux, 2006; Powell et al., 2007, and Zenk et al., 2006. Moreover, research suggests that lower income and non-white communities (demographic groups at increased risk for overweight and obesity) are more likely to have reduced access to nutritious and affordable food (Morland et al., 2002; Moore & Diez Roux, 2006; Zenk et al., 2005, 2006).

Macro Environment

Pricing/Economics

Yet another influence on Americans' dietary behavior may be economic. According to Lakdawalla and Philipson (2002), the relative price of food has decreased substantially over the last several decades, and that simple supply and demand has increased consumption. Similarly, Bleich, Cutler, Murray and Adamis (2007) found that decreased food prices corresponded to increased caloric supply. In addition, Cutler, Glaeser and Shapiro (2003) argued that recent technological advances have lowered the costs of obtaining food, and this has contributed to the rise in obesity rates. Drewnowski and Specter (2004) have argued that energy-dense, nutritionally-poor food is cheaper than healthier options, which encourages consumption of high-calorie food choices.

Media/Advertising

Advertising for energy-dense/nutritionally-poor food may also contribute to its over-consumption (Story et al., 2001). Children appear particularly vulnerable to advertising and below eight years of age, cannot discriminate the persuasive intent of marketing—that is, the difference between information and advertising (Koplan et al., 2005; McGinnis et al., 2005). The food and beverage industry spends approximately $10-12 billion annually on marketing to children and teens in the United States, most of which is for high calorie/low nutrient foods and beverages (McGinnis et al., 2005; Nestle, 2003). A 2005 report by the IOM concluded that there was strong evidence that television advertising influenced the food and beverage preferences and purchase requests of children 2-11 years of age, as well as strong evidence that television advertising was associated with overweight in children and teens aged 2-18 (McGinnis et al., 2005).

Overall, there does not appear to be a simple or single cause for rapidly rising obesity rates. Rather, increased obesity prevalence is linked to a number of environmental changes that have occurred at multiple levels of the social-ecological model. The following section briefly reviews the research approach of this dissertation

Summary of Research Approach

This dissertation examines obesity in the context of market failure. The research question examined is: *What are the lifetime, external costs of a 1000-person obese cohort in the United States, in comparison to one of normal weight?* Based (1) conceptually on the studies by Manning et al. (1989, 1991) and Keeler et al. (1989) on the lifetime, external costs of smoking, excessive alcohol consumption and lack of physical activity, and (2) methodologically on a study by Tucker et al. (2006) that modeled obesity-related costs such as healthcare and quality of life, this dissertation develops a model of the lifetime external costs of obesity in two phases. Phase One surveys and summarizes the costing literature on obesity to inform cost categories and estimates. Phase Two develops a Markov model using inputs from Phase One and the literature review, to calculate net present value of the lifetime, external costs of a normal weight cohort versus those of an obese cohort.

The dissertation proceeds as follows: Chapter Two reviews the obesity-related economic literature and locates this dissertation within that context. Chapter Three details this dissertation's methodology. Chapter Four reports on the results of the analysis conducted for this dissertation. Chapter Five discusses the policy implications of the findings reported here, describes limitations and contributions of this study, and summarizes the dissertation.

Conclusion

This chapter examined the background on this issue of obesity—its trends, health and economic effects, and causes/correlates—and provided summary details of the research question and methods of this dissertation. In brief, obesity rates in the United States have increased dramatically in the last several decades, particularly since the late 1970s and early 1980s. Obesity prevalence has increased in adults and in children, and racial and ethnic minorities are at increased risk for overweight and obesity. However, the association between SES and obesity is not consistent. Obesity affects mortality and

morbidity risks, and obesity is a risk factor for several forms of cancer, diabetes type 2,

coronary heart disease, gallstones, osteoarthritis and many other health conditions.

Although genetics are a significant factor in the development of overweight and obesity,

the rapid population-level increase in obesity cannot be explained by genetics and

biology alone. Instead, environmental factors across the social-ecological model are

implicated. Many of these factors may be addressed by policymakers. The following

chapter reviews the economic literature related to obesity.

Chapter Two: Literature Review

Introduction

Having examined the background on the issue of obesity, this chapter reviews and locates

the present study within the economics literature on obesity. A conceptual diagram of

these literatures is provided in Figure 2.1. In comparison to the work on obesity from

public health and biomedicine, the economic literature on obesity is relatively sparse. For

example, searching on the term *obes** (where * is a wildcard) in **abstracts** in EconLit, a

search engine which indexes economic literature, returned 163 articles, whereas

searching on *obesity* in the **title** in the Web of Science search engine returned more than

100,000 articles.[3]

Figure 2.1: Conceptual Diagram of Literature Reviewed

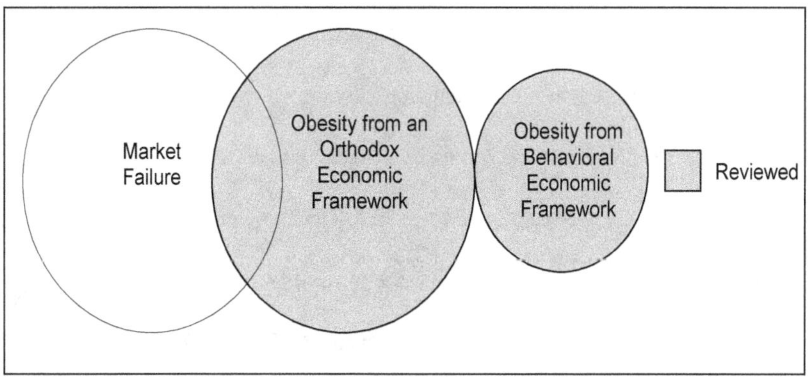

There are four main sections of this chapter: (1) key economic concepts and assumptions;

(2) economic literature on obesity and the market failure; (3) obesity-related literature

---

[3] Search conducted on 9/15/2007

from an "orthodox" economic framework; (4) the small literature on obesity from a behavioral economic frame. These four areas are reviewed in turn in the sections that follow.

Key Economic Concepts and Assumptions

Market Failure

According to "neoclassical" (used synonymously throughout this dissertation with the terms "standard" and "orthodox") economics, the decisions of rational, well-informed individuals collectively form the "invisible hand" of the market. The market then allocates scarce societal resources in a Pareto efficient manner (Bator, 1958), i.e., where no one person may be made better off without making another worse off. However, the market may fail to distribute these resources efficiently, which is termed "market failure". For Bator (1958), who was among the earliest to discuss the concept, market failure is "the failure of a more or less idealized system of price-market institutions to sustain 'desirable' activities or to stop 'undesirable' activities" (p. 351). "Activities" in this case refer both to production and consumption. Similarly, Friedman (2002) describes market failures as "situations in which ordinary market coordination does not lead to an efficient (perfectly competitive) equilibrium" (p. 593). The following are examples of market failure: public goods, externalities, market power (monopoly/oligopoly) and information failure (Friedman, 2002; Office of Management and Budget [OMB], 2003; Weimer & Vining, 2005).

Within welfare economics, the existence of serious market failure provides the rationale for government intervention (Calwey, 2004; Friedman, 2002; OMB, 2003; Weimer & Vining, 2005). Evidence that supports or weakens the argument for market failure as it relates to obesity is therefore central to this dissertation.

Consumer Sovereignty

"Consumer sovereignty" is the belief that individuals are the most effective judges of their own best interest. As Friedman (2002) states: "consumer sovereignty means that each person is the sole judge of his or her own welfare" (p.46). Economics as a discipline generally assumes a generous view of individuals' capacity to judge their own best interests.

Rationality

The concept of rationality is intrinsic to the notion of consumer sovereignty. Rationality in an economic sense means that an individual is *capable* of judging his or her own best interests, not whether or not one actually *agrees* with their assessment. Many people undertake activities that others might deem too risky and would not undertake (e.g., mountain-climbing or hang-gliding). Yet, from an economic frame of reference they should be allowed to participate in these activities, as long as they bear the associated costs and are aware of the risks. Further, it is generally agreed that individuals are not "perfectly rational" and do not possess perfect knowledge and perfect cognitive abilities. Instead, as described by Herbert Simon (1955), individuals are limited in their ability to access and process information, and make rational decisions within their capacity to store, retrieve and process information. That is, individuals are "boundedly rational".

Other Assumptions

Economists also assume that health is not a person's only goal; they believe that individuals seek to maximize their utility, within constraints such as income, time, sleep, and others. Individuals are therefore viewed as producers of their own health (Connelly, 2004), within certain constraints. Economists such as Grossman and Cawley have described models of individual health production (Cawley, 2004; Grossman, 1972). Michael Grossman's seminal work provides an early model in which health is a function of one's initial health stock (basic biology), as well as medical care, lifestyle, environment, income and education. Cawley (2004) developed the SLOTH model of time allocation, where health and weight are the result of a person's utility maximization function, according to time spent pursing the following activities: Sleep, Leisure, Occupation, Transportation, and Home production, and their genetic makeup, which determines metabolic rate.

Economists also assume that people make conscious decisions related to dietary behavior, and that in the process of deciding what to eat, individuals evaluate short and long term effects of their decisions. As Cawley (2004) notes: "When deciding whether to eat large amounts of saturated fat, skip vegetables, be sedentary… individuals weigh the utility benefits of the behavior (e.g., taste, relaxation) against the welfare losses of the behavior (e.g., higher risk of morbidity or mortality). Economists accept that people may rationally choose to participate in an activity that increases morbidity or mortality" (p.118). In this way, many economists consider overweight and obesity a choice, as evidenced by this passage from Philipson (2001):

> More than many physical conditions, obesity is avoidable by behavioral changes, which economists expect to be undertaken if the benefits exceed the costs… In a rational-choice model… there is no such thing as 'overweight'. Weight is the result of personal choices along such dimensions as occupation, leisure-time activity or inactivity, residence, and, of course, food intake. Being either fat or thin may therefore be as desirable from the individual's standpoint as adhering to the norms to the norms of weight set by doctors and the public health community. (p.1)

Economic Literature on Obesity as Market Failure and Government Intervention
Having reviewed some key concepts and assumptions relevant to this dissertation, this section examines the literature on obesity as market failure. Economists generally discuss obesity as an example of market failure in the context of externalities, information failure and imperfect rationality. These categories are reviewed in turn in the sections that follow. There is little consensus among economists on whether increased obesity prevalence constitutes an example of market failure, as evidenced by the following quotations:

> Americans' rapid weight gain may have nothing to do with market failure. It may be the rational response to changing technology and prices… So, if consumers willingly trade off increased adiposity for working indoors and

spending less time in the kitchen as well as for manageable weight-related

health problems, then markets are not failing. (Kuchler, Golan, Variyam,

& Crutchfield, 2005, p.30)

But—obese people only hurt themselves—right? If that is true, then from

an economic standpoint people should be at liberty to make any diet and

exercise choices they wish, including those which place them at greater

risk of becoming obese. (Elston, Stanton, Levy, & Acs, 2007, p.172)

There is a strong, logical argument that there is an externality associated

with obesity, although this has not been unequivocally proven…

Similarly, it is likely that there are significant gaps in information which

would justify government intervention… There appears to be a strong *a*

priori case for government intervention to protect children. (McCormick,

et al., 2007, p.164)

Obesity and Externalities

There has been little empirical work to date on the externalities linked with obesity. As

Cawley (2004) notes, the exceptions to this include the work of Finkelstein et al. (2003),

which determined the annual cost to publicly funded healthcare programs of obesity, and

the work of Keeler et al. (1989) which calculated the financial externalities associated

with sedentary behavior. In contrast, most of the discussion in the literature on obesity

and the existence of externalities is conjecture. These discussions largely center on the

financial externalities of obesity, although the health externalities of obesity are also briefly mentioned. The absence of lifetime costing models has hindered calculation of

externalities. This dissertation and the development of a lifetime model of external costs

responds to this gap in the literature. The work on externalities and obesity largely falls

into the category of financial externalities, although Finkelstein & Zuckerman (2008) also

discuss the negative health effects of obese mothers during pregnancy on their children as

an externality that justifies government intervention.

Financial Externalities

Several researchers have previously speculated that the financial externalities related to

the healthcare costs associated with obesity may constitute an example of market failure

and therefore provide a rationale for government intervention (Anderson, Butcher, &

Levine, 2003b; Cawley, 2007; Elston et al., 2007; Kuchler et al., 2005; McCormick et al.,

2007). Kuchler et al. (2005) observe that consumers often do not bear the full financial

costs of their dietary and physical activity decisions due to current healthcare insurance

practices. Therefore, to the extent that taxpayers (e.g., for Medicare and Medicaid

participants) and others in an insurance risk pool pay through their employers, this may

be considered an example of market failure. McCormick et al. (2007), writing of the

experience of the United Kingdom, also note that full healthcare costs may not be borne

by the obese individual.

Cawley (2007) discusses the financial externalities of healthcare costs in general terms,

referencing earlier costing studies by Finkelstein (2003) and life insurance costs, but

notes the possibility of *positive* financial externalities of obesity:

On the other hand, to the extent that obese or sedentary individuals

participate in defined-benefit pension plans and tend to die younger than

or more active people, they generate positive externalities because they die

before they can collect their full share of pension benefits. Likewise,

obese individuals may on average draw fewer social security benefits.

(p.40)

Elston et al., (2007) discuss the existence of financial externalities associated with obesity

in general terms, noting that if obesity is the result of individual decision-making and

only affects the individual, then there is no justification for government intervention.

Citing previous costing studies, Elston et al. conclude however, that the external costs

imposed on society broadly by obese individuals justifies government intervention:

"Thus, obesity generates negative externalities. In other words, obesity does not just

affect the obese but those who bear the costs of others' obesity through public programs,

risk pooling, collectively financed programs and other sources." (p.175)

McCormick et al. (2007) discuss the financial externalities associated with obesity

beyond healthcare costs, noting that obese individuals are more likely to be unemployed,

and while the individual loses wages, society is also impacted in lower tax revenues and

increased unemployment benefits. McCormick et al. (2007) further observe that the

lifetime costs versus the most immediate costs are not known at this point, and therefore

the financial externalities obesity are not clear.

Obesity and Information Failure

The existence of information-failure is also debated within the literature on market failure and obesity, and falls into three broad areas: under-provision of information; adverse selection; and false or misleading information. The following subsections discuss these areas in turn.

Under-Provision of Information

Information relevant to obesity may be under-provided in three main areas: the benefits associated with improved/poor diet and increased physical activity; an individual's weight status and personal risk; and lack of information regarding the nutritional content of food.

In the first area—knowledge about the beneficial effects of a healthy diet and regular physical activity—Cawley (2004) says that information is "underprovided and disseminated" by government sources, noting the huge disparity between food and beverage manufacturers' marketing budgets, relative to the US federal government budget for the 5-A-Day (now "Fruit and Veggies: More Matters") campaign to increase fruit and vegetable consumption. In this case, objective information may be costly for the consumer to source and use, and will likely be used only when marginal benefits outweigh costs. Cawley further asserts that not only is more information needed, but that it should be provided in a form that consumers can use easily.

In contrast, Finkelstein and Zuckerman (2008) argue against under-provision of information as an example of market failure with regard to obesity, noting the regular publication of dietary guidelines for Americans, nutrition labeling requirements on packaged food, the increased NIH budget for obesity research; and CDC and federal government grants and activities provide ample information for consumers. In addition, Kuchler et al. (2005) comment that the overwhelming volume of media coverage about weight and diet suggests that Americans should be well informed about the linkage between healthy diet and its protective effect against overweight.

In the second area of potential under-provision of information—knowledge of personal risk—Kuchler et al. (2005) speculate about the possibility that Americans are not aware of their own weight status and/or risk. According to their report for the USDA Economic Research Service (ERS), Kuchler et al. state that 41 percent of persons classified as overweight did not perceive themselves to be so, and that 13 percent of technically obese persons thought their weight was low to normal.

The third area where information may be underprovided relates to the nutritional content of food. It is possible that individuals may unknowingly consume excess calories. As mentioned in Chapter One, consumers have increased their consumption of food away from home in the last several decades, yet often nutritional information about that food is not readily available. Cawley (2004) notes that that nutrition labels affect people's behavior, but restaurant food in particular does not provide nutrition information for the consumer. In addition, Kuchler et al. (2005) cite the lack of available nutrition information in restaurants as possible evidence of market failure, noting that in a 1996 study, even dieticians were unable to estimate correctly the caloric and fat content of meals in restaurants, and underestimated these by considerable amounts in both cases.

Adverse Selection

Cawley (2007) discusses the possibility of adverse selection in health insurance among obese individuals as an example of information-failure, where obese participants choose to participate in programs that cover obesity treatment such as weight-loss programs. This may lead to higher premiums, reducing participation among normal weight participants, causing a 'premium death spiral'. Cawley notes however that the impact of adverse selection on the health insurance market in this case is not currently known.

Misleading Information

In the last example obesity as information-failure, Cawley (2004) observes that some information provided by the private sector is misleading. For example, labeling vegetable oil as 'cholesterol free' (when it is inherently so) may imply to some consumers that it may be particularly beneficial.

Obesity and Imperfect Rationality

Imperfect rationality is the third area where increased obesity prevalence may be an example of market failure. The assumption of rational actors is a core underpinning of orthodox economics, as noted earlier. A lack of rationality by individuals may therefore justify government intervention, and several economists discuss imperfect rationality as a possible example of market failure with regard to the issue of obesity (Anderson et al., 2003b; Calwley 2004; McCormick et al., 2007; Moodie, Swinburn, Richardson, & Somainin, 2006). The discussion in the literature on rationality in the context of obesity largely centers on children, although is also discussed with regard to adults, sometimes in the context of addiction.

Imperfect Rationality and Children

Several researchers cite children as examples of imperfectly rational actors in the context of obesity-related market failure (Anderson et al., 2003b; Cawley, 2007; Cawley, 2004; McCormick et al., Moodie et al., 2006). As Cawley (2004) observes, it is generally accepted that children are incapable of fully accounting for the consequences of their actions. Further, there is ample precedent for restrictions with regard to children and teens—e.g., banning sales of cigarettes and alcohol to youth.

Imperfect Rationality and Adults

McCormick et al. (2007) describe "protecting vulnerable individuals" as another form of market failure and rationale for government intervention. This term refers to lack of rationality, as in the case of both children, and addictive goods. McCormick et al. explain this as follows: "In this case, food, or weight more generally, might be regarded as a type of demerit good in which (at least some) individuals are unable to be an optimal judge of their own welfare". (p.163)

Moodie et al. (2006) question the rationality of some consumers as a basis for market failure: "People may not have the… analytical ability, strength of character, or will to convert what they know to be best for themselves or their children into effective action" (p.136). McCormick et al. (2007) also question the rationality of some food behavior, noting that some food has been described as addictive, or that some people may have self-control issues. In some cases, people may behave in a way where their preferences are inconsistent over time, for example their need for instant gratification outweighs their long-term preferences. According to Cutler et al. (2003), at least some food consumption is not rational.

Other Orthodox Economic Literature on Obesity

Other orthodox economic literature related to obesity falls into the following three main categories: (1) Costs, for example healthcare and other societal costs of obesity; (2) Correlates and causal influences of obesity prevalence; and (3) Other analyses of specific phenomena relevant to obesity.

The first area, costs, will be discussed in detail in Chapter Four, as the purpose of Phase One of this dissertation's methodology is to locate and report on the relevant costing studies related to obesity. However, a review of the lifetime costing studies is provided here, as these are the studies most akin to this dissertation. Allison, Zannoli, and Narayan (1999) and Thompson, Edelsberg, Colditz, Bird, and Oster (1999) calculated lifetime costs using population attributable risk (PAR) methodology. PAR uses the costs of obesity-related individual diseases, such as diabetes type 2, then estimates the proportion of these costs due to obesity. PAR methodology limits the number of diseases in its cost calculations, however, and may not account for duplicate costs of co-morbidities. Tucker et al. (2006) used Monte Carlo simulations to assess a mixture of internal and external costs, including healthcare and quality of life. Finkelstein et al. (2008) used economic modeling to assess lifetime costs of healthcare. Lakdawalla, Goldman, and Shang (2005), and Daviglus et al. (2004) both assessed healthcare costs related to the Medicare population.

The second area of orthodox economic literature related to obesity—correlates and causal influences—has been woven into the section on causal influences in Chapter One, which includes work stemming from the field of public health as well as economics. As a brief review, these economic studies relate to several areas of the social-ecological model of eating and physical activity behavior and include: the association between restaurants and obesity Chou, Grossman, & Saffer, 2002, 2004; Rashad, Grossman, & Chou, 2006); the effect of advances in technology which alter costs associated with eating and physical activity behavior (Bleich et al., 2007; Cutler et al., 2003; Lakdawalla & Philipson, 2002; Popkin et al., 2006); food assistance and agricultural subsidies (Asfaw, 2007; Kaushall, 2007; Miller & Coble, 2007); individual-level influences such as genetics, and social interactions (Costa-Font & Gil, 2004); advertising (Anderson & Butcher, 2006b) and finally the effect of the built environment (Eid et al., 2007; Plantinga & Bernell, 2005). Researchers have also found links between reduced tobacco use and increased rates of obesity (Chou et al., 2002, 2004; Rashad et al., 2006), although a causal connection between the two was not supported by the research of Gruber and Frakes (2006).

The third main areas of orthodox economic literature on obesity focuses on analysis of particular phenomena associated with obesity. These phenomena include: the effect of obesity on wages/employment; education, SES and participation in the Food Stamp Program (FSP) (now known at the Supplemental Nutrition Assistance Program or SNAP); health and health insurance; and other analyses. The following sections survey these literatures.

Obesity and Wages/Employment

Several studies show an inverse relationship between wages and obesity (Averett & Korenman, 1996; Baum & Ford, 2004; Bhattacharya & Sood, 2005b; Pagan & Davila, 1997; Zagorsky, 2005). However, the cause(s) of this association is debated. Pagan and Davlia (1997), Averett and Korenman (1996), and Baum and Ford (2004) hypothesize that the wage differential between obese and normal weight persons may be due to labor discrimination. For example, Baum and Ford studied the effect of obesity on earnings using National Longitudinal Survey of Youth (NLSY) data, and found a persistent wage effect in the first 20 years of a person's career of 0.7 to 6.3 percent. This effect was not explained by SES or other family-related variables, suggesting labor discrimination may be the cause. Bhattacharya and Bundorf (2005a) also found evidence of such a wage effect, but found that it may be a compensatory effect for the higher healthcare costs incurred by the obese, and not due to labor discrimination in fulltime workers with pooled health insurance.

This wage effect between obese and normal weight persons appears to vary according to race and gender. Averett and Korenman (1996), Pagan and Davila (1997), Zagorsky (2005), Cawley and Danziger (2005) and Bhattacharya and Bundorf (2005a) found that the wage differential between obese and non-obese workers greater in women than men. Moreover, this effect seemed far stronger in whites than African Americans. Averett and Korenman found that obese African American women did not appear to earn lower wages relative to other African American women, and Zagorsky found there was a large negative effect on wealth for white women, which was smaller in black women and white men, and no relationship between wealth and weight in black men. Cawley and Danziger examined the relationship between morbid obesity and transitioning between welfare and employment, and found that morbidly obese white women were adversely affected; they spend longer on welfare and receive lower wages when working. No such differential on labor outcomes was found in African American women.

Education, SES, Food Assistance and Obesity

Several studies have examined the association between obesity, and factors such as education, SES and food assistance, although it is likely there is a high degree of confounding between these factors and BMI. Mancino, Lin, & Ballenger (2004) found that socioeconomic factors "significantly and systematically affect an individual's ability to achieve good health" (p. iii). Sabia (2007) examined the connection between BMI and academic performance in teens, and found evidence of a causal connection in white girls, but not in white boys, or other races/ethnicities. Nayga (2000, 2001) studied the association between education, health knowledge and obesity, and found that schooling was inversely associated with BMI, although it appeared that this was due to increased health knowledge, rather than schooling itself. However, Kenkel, Lillard and Mathios (2006) did not find a relationship between high-school graduation (or obtaining a Graduate Equivalency Degree) and obesity, in contrast to other public health studies of obesity.

Baum and Ruhm (2007) investigated the development of obesity over one's lifetime, and its relationship to SES. Similar to other findings, Baum found that weight was inversely related to SES, but that a large amount of the correlation between SES and weight may be explained by race/ethnicity, family background, and its impact on education. Boumtje, Huang, Lee, & Lin, (2005) also found evidence of an association between overweight and poverty in children in an investigation of a range of factors associated with obesity. Researchers report conflicting findings with respect to participation in the food stamp program (FSP) and its effect on bodyweight. Chen, Yen, & Eastwood, (2005) found a positive association between FSP participation and obesity in women, but not for men. In contrast, Ver Ploeg, Mancino, Lin, & Wang, (2007) found that a significant association existed between FSP participation and obesity in the 1976-1981 NHANES survey data—particularly amongst white women—but that association no longer existed in the 2000-2002 survey, which may have resulted from the general population increase in BMI.

Health or Health Insurance- Related Topics

Several economists have examined obesity with respect to health or health insurance. Vandegrift and Datta (2006) studied spending on prescription drugs in the United States

1990-98, and found that 8% of the 84% increase in drug spending in this period was due to obesity. Rashad and Markowitz (2007) investigated the possible influence of health insurance on weight, but did not find that existence of health insurance exerted a causal influence on the likelihood of being obese. Cutler and Glaeser (2007) studied the health profile of the US population and found that it has generally improved due to reduced smoking and better control of blood pressure. Obesity does not appear to have substantially increased mortality risk to date, however Cutler predicts that this will change in the next 20 years. Finally, Kan and Tsai (2004) examined the association between knowledge of health risks and obesity, and found that a relationship existed in men who were extremely overweight, but was not significantly associated with BMI in women.

Other Economic Analyses

Other economic analyses of obesity-related issues cover a diverse range of topics, including the Nutrition Labeling and Education Act (NLEA), obesity prevalence projections, using BMI as a measure of adiposity, physical education regulations, time preference, the Americans with Disabilities Act, and the responsiveness of consumers to changes in food prices. This sub-section briefly reports on these studies and their findings.

Nutrition Labeling and Education Act

Variyam and Cawley (2006) examined the effects of changes to the NLEA. They found

that use of the labels was largely restricted to non-Hispanic white women, but for that

group, using the labels correlated to decreases in bodyfat.

Obesity Prevalence Projections

Ruhm (2007), using NHANES data, projected obesity and severe obesity levels through

2020.

Other Measures of Adiposity

Cawley (2006b) examined the effect of not using BMI as the measure for obesity. In this

particular study, Cawley provided conversions from BMI to other measures, such as total

bodyfat, percent bodyfat, and waist to hip ratio. Cawley estimated reduced prevalence of

obesity in African American men and women using these other measures of adiposity.

Relationship between Time Preference and Weight

Smith, Bogin and Bishai (2005) studied the relationship between time preference (the rate

a person will trade future for current utility) and weight by using a proxy measure of

willingness to save. In the case of obesity, these tradeoffs include short-term enjoyment

of food against long-term health effects. Smith et al. found evidence of a significant

relationship between time preference and weight in black and Hispanic men and in black

women. Carpenter (2006) examined the effect of a court case Cook v Rhode Island and the Americans with Disabilities Act on the labor market, and found that the case

increased employment 4% for obese women and 2% for obese men.

Price Elasticity

Finally, there is research on the effects of price changes on food consumption. Kuchler,

Tegene, and Harris (2004), investigated the effect of taxing salty snacks on consumption.

They found that low tax rates (in the order of 1%) did not change consumption

substantially, but their analysis revealed it may produce tax revenue in the range of $40-

100 million. Huang and Lin (2000) developed household estimates of elasticities for food

and nutrients, based on 1987-8 Nationwide Food Consumption Survey (NFCS).

In summary, the neoclassical economic literature related to obesity falls into three overall

categories: costs, correlates and causal influences, and analysis of particular phenomena,

such as the relationship between obesity and wages/employment. We now turn to an

examination of behavioral economic literature and obesity

Behavioral Economics and Obesity Literature

This section reviews the small literature of behavioral economic research and obesity.

Although relatively little research exists in this area, the work that has been done may

have implications for possible public policy interventions. This section provides

background information on the differences between behavioral and orthodox economics,

then reviews the literature on obesity from a behavioral economic frame. The work that

has been completed in behavioral economics and obesity largely concern experiments on food choice and physical activity behavior in adults and children, and more recently, work on food assistance programs and their implications for policy.

Introduction to Behavioral Economics

Behavioral economics is a relatively new branch of economics that blends microeconomic concepts and rational choice models with the experimental methods and perspectives of psychology (Epstein, 1998; Madden, 2000; Just 2006). For Madden (2000), "[t]ogether these techniques and principles are employed to gain a more complete understanding of the interaction between behavior and the economic context in which it occurs" (p.6.). According to Just (2006), behavioral economic concepts and application has been embraced most fully by researchers interested in issues of finance. Behavioral economics differs from the standard economic frame in several ways, including the use of individual, experimental data rather than population-level data, and its treatment of rationality. Just (2006) notes that "[b]ehavioral economists have found that individuals tend to deviate from what is often termed rational behavior in highly systematic and predictable ways" (p. 210). According to Thaler and Sunstein (2003):

> People do not exhibit rational expectations, fail to make forecasts that are
> consistent with Bayes' rule, use heuristics that lead them to make
> systematic blunders, exhibit preference reversals (that is, they prefer A to
> B and B to A) and make different choices depending on the wording of the
> problem... Furthermore, in the context of intertemporal choice, people
> exhibit dynamic inconsistency, valuing present consumption much more

than future consumption. In other words, people have self-control

problems." (p.176)

In addition, behavioral economists draw from neuroscience in distinguishing between

two kinds of thinking: 1) Reflexive/automatic, and 2) Reflective/deliberative (Thaler and

Sunstein, 2008).

For some, behavioral economics extends rational choice theory (Epstein, 1998), whereas

others see it as allowing "departures from rationality" (Cawley, 2007, p. 32). As an

example related to the issue of rationality, several studies in behavioral finance on 401(k)

plans have shown that default options matter a great deal (Choi, Laibson, & Madrien

2002; Madrien & Shea, 2001), yet if the actors were fully rational, defaults should not

matter. If enrolled automatically in a plan, a small percentage of participants opt out.

However if not automatically enrolled, only around 50% of eligible participants will

choose to participate in the plan (Choi, Laibson, Madrian, & Metrick, 2003).

Obesity-Related Behavioral Economics: Diet and Physical Activity Behavior

The behavioral economics literature on obesity is relatively small, although there is a

more extensive literature of diet and physical activity decision-making that is not

reviewed here. Instead, this section summarizes the behavioral economic research

directly related to obesity. This behavioral economic literature suggests that humans'

dietary and physical activity behavior may not be fully rational. This imperfect rationality

has implications for obesity-related public policy interventions, which is discussed in

Chapter Five.

Several authors have examined behavioral economic choices with regard to eating and physical activity in obese subjects (Smith & Epstein, 1991; Lappalianen & Epstein (1990); Saelens & Epstein 1998, 1996). In an experiment on obese children, Smith and Epstein (1991) found that responses to preference schedules differed between highly liked foods, moderately liked foods and the work required to obtain them. Their results showed that children were strongly influenced by environmental factors, such as price and distance the food outlet, as well as how much they liked the food choices. Children switched to moderately liked foods when the effort required to obtain the more highly preferred foods increased beyond a certain level.

Epstein and Saelens (2000) reviewed the behavioral economics literature on food choice (i.e., what to eat and how much) and levels of physical activity in the context of obesity. The review suggests that food choice and levels of physical activity are strongly influenced by the way constraints are imposed or healthy behaviors are reinforced. This work indicates preferences for certain foods in addition to environmental constraints will affect food choice. For example, a food liked less than a more desirable (high in fat and sugar) choice will be chosen if the latter is less accessible—i.e., the cost for its consumption is increased. Additionally, the convenience of physical activity appears to influence activity levels. The rate at which children and adults substitute to healthier food and physical activity choices away from less healthy choices by increasing work required were not uniform, but rather varied by obesity level (normal weight, overweight or obese). Overall, this may offer some insight on how behavior has changed at the population level as our environment provides ready access to highly desirable (high

calorie) food, and decreased requirement for physical activity.

Obesity-Related Behavioral Economics: Supplemental Nutrition Programs

Research on the USDA nutrition supplement programs suggests that eating behavior

among beneficiaries departs from rationality as understood in standard economics. These

programs impact a large number of Americans (Just, Mancino, & Wansink, 2007). The

largest programs include the Supplemental Nutrition Assistance Program (SNAP), the

Special Supplemental Nutrition Program for Women, Infants, and Children, (WIC), and

the National School Lunch and School Breakfast Programs. Some research analyzes food

stamp recipients' behavior to assess ways in which food assistance may be redesigned

(Just et al., 2007; Just, 2006). Just et al. (2007) note that dietary behavior in food stamp

recipients conflicts with standard economic assumptions: food stamp recipients often

spend their benefits and some additional cash on food. However, if provided with a cash

equivalent, recipients will spend less overall on food. In another example, food stamp

beneficiaries often front-load their spending on food after receiving benefits, then may

have little to no food at the end of the benefit period. This suggests a level of future

discounting beyond standard economic assumptions.

Another USDA report examined eating behavior from a behavioral economics

perspective. Findings in the report support the notion that food decisions depart from a

rational calculation of costs and benefits. Rather, eating appears to be based on emotional decisions, subject to influences such as external cues, including portion sizes, and "default options", such as more healthful school menu defaults (Just et al., 2007).

Conclusion

This chapter surveyed the economic literature on obesity as market failure, in addition to the literatures on obesity from orthodox and behavioral economic frames. The following key points emerged: First, the economic literature on obesity is relatively small, which is somewhat surprising, given the extent of the issue and its potential impact in economic terms. Second, there is little agreement amongst economists regarding whether obesity constitutes an example of market failure. Third, the discussions regarding market failure and obesity have fallen into the categories of financial externalities, information-failure and imperfect rationality. Fourth, the economic literature related to obesity falls into the following topic areas: costs; causal influences; and analyses of specific phenomena such as the impact of obesity on wages, or the effects of small taxes on food consumption. Lastly, behavioral economics may offer some insights on diet and physical activity behavior, which may be important in any possible policy interventions.

Significantly, for the purposes of this dissertation, little empirical work exists on the financial externalities related to obesity. A calculation of the lifetime, external costs of obesity fills an important gap in the literature, and may contribute to the debate on obesity as market failure. Having reviewed the economic literature relevant to obesity, the next chapter outlines this dissertation's methodology.

Chapter Three: Methods

Introduction

This chapter describes the methodology of the analysis undertaken for this dissertation. As noted in Chapter Two, financial externalities appear to be one of several possible examples of market failure associated with obesity. Many have estimated individual component costs of obesity, e.g., healthcare costs, quality of life, and costs to businesses. However, a rigorous estimation of the net present value, lifetime, external costs of obesity has not been undertaken. Such an estimate fills an important gap in the literature, and may inform the debate regarding potential policy interventions. Results of the analysis described here are provided in Chapter Four.

The present study was inspired conceptually by Manning et al. (1989, 1991) and Keeler et al. (1989), and methodologically by Tucker et al. (2006). In 1989 and 1991, Manning, Keeler and colleagues published seminal articles and a book estimating the external costs of smoking, heavy drinking and lack of exercise using economic modeling. These works included: "The Taxes of Sin: Do Smokers and Drinkers Pay Their Way?" in the *Journal of the American Medical Association* (Manning et al., 1989); "The External Cost of a Sedentary Lifestyle, in the *American Journal of Public Health* (Keeler et al., 1989) and the book *The Costs of Poor Health Habits* (Manning et al., 1991). In these studies, researchers developed hypothetical 1000-person cohorts with and without the health behavior in question, and compared the cohorts' lifetime, external costs from age 20 to

64

age 85 or death, whichever came first. Many of the costs used in these analyses were sources from primary data gathered during the RAND health experiment[4] (Manning et al. 1989). In contrast, Tucker et al. (2006) used micro-simulation techniques to estimate lifetime costs of obesity related to healthcare and quality of life for hypothetical 1000-person cohorts, using published data sources: "Counting the Costs of Overweight and Obesity: Modeling Clinical and Cost Outcomes" in *Current Medical Research and Opinion.*

Lacking access to similar primary data sources available to the researchers in the Manning et al. studies, and given that many researchers have already carefully estimated individual component costs of obesity such as healthcare costs, the methodology of this dissertation proceeds in the following two phases:

1) <u>Phase One: A meta-analysis of existing obesity costing research.</u> This first phase identifies and summarizes published obesity costing literature. Generally, studies in this area focus on estimating costs of a specific aspect of obesity, such as healthcare costs. The meta-analysis serves two key functions: First, it identifies many of the cost areas associated with obesity. Second, it provides the basis for the costing inputs for several of the lifetime cost estimates in Phase Two.

2) <u>Phase Two: An analysis of the external costs of obesity.</u> The second phase calculates the costs to society of obesity, based on several of the cost-estimates derived from Phase One. This study creates a Markov model of two hypothetical 20 year-old, demographically representative, 1000-person

---

[4] For more information on the Rand Health Experiment, see Rand (2008)

cohorts, one obese, the other normal weight. These cohorts are then 'aged'

using simulation software until age 85 or death, whichever comes first. The

resulting differences in external costs between the cohorts are then calculated

by the software.

This chapter details the methodology by which an estimate of obesity's external costs

were determined, and is divided into two main sections. The first section explains the

process by which the meta-analysis of existing obesity costing literature was undertaken,

including search terms, search engines and inclusion/exclusion criteria. The second

section details how the computer simulation model was created to estimate the net

present value of the lifetime, external costs of obesity.

Phase One: Meta-Analysis of the Obesity Costing Literature

The first phase of the methodology in this dissertation serves to locate, summarize and

review the relevant literature on the costing of obesity. This review provides the basis for

several of the cost estimates in phase two by: 1) establishing the external costing

categories for obesity such as healthcare; and 2) providing dollar cost estimates for the

individual external components needed in Phase Two. The search and inclusion/exclusion

criteria for this synthesis review are reviewed in the following section.

Search and Inclusion/Exclusion Criteria

The following key search terms were used to locate relevant obesity costing articles in the

peer-reviewed literature: cost*, economic*, social, obesity, "cost estimate," healthcare, absenteeism, disability, "cost estimates," "social cost," and "cost of illness." The search engines used to locate the articles included: ISI Web of Science, Scopus, ProQuest Research Library Plus, and EconLit. A search was also conducted of authors who have been widely cited for their work on obesity costing, including Eric Finkelstein, Anne Wolf, Graham Colditz and David Thompson. In addition, a "snowball method" was used, whereby references in articles located using the search criteria were also examined and included, where appropriate.

Articles included in the meta-analysis were limited to those that assess obesity costs and have been published in peer-reviewed journals from January, 1990 to October, 2008. Healthcare costing studies were limited to those assessments of United States healthcare costs. Studies from other countries that address costs other than healthcare have been included to provide context, but their cost estimates were not used in the model developed in Phase Two. Articles that have been excluded from the final compilation include: abstracts, costing studies on individual illnesses (such as type 2 diabetes), and quality of life studies. The results of the meta-analysis are provided in Chapter Four. Having described the meta-analysis of obesity-related costing studies, the following section describes how the external costs associated with obesity were calculated.

Phase Two: Markov Model of Net, External, Lifetime Obesity Costs

Overview

Phase Two of the methodology in this dissertation is the development of a Markov model to estimate the net present value of the lifetime, external costs related to obesity. The

Markov model was created using simulation software: TreeAge Pro 2009 (TreeAge

Software Inc., Williamstown, Massachusetts, http://www.treeage.com/). Using TreeAge,

two hypothetical, demographically representative of the U.S., 1000-person, obese and

normal weight cohorts were created. These cohorts were then "aged" from 20 to 85 years

or death, and the external costs associated with obesity compared. The 1000-person

cohorts are racially/ethnically diverse (including non-Hispanic whites, non-Hispanic

blacks and Hispanics) and include both sexes. The proportions for these racial/ethnic and

gender-based groups are described in a later section on cohort demographics. BMI for the

obese cohort starts at a range intended to be representative of obesity levels in 20-year

olds in the United States, and BMI then varies over each cohort member's "lifetime".

Lifetables developed by Fontaine et al. (2003) are used to assess the weight-related

probability of death. Figure 3.1 provides a graphical representation of the obese cohort

developed in TreeAge, with most of the sub-trees collapsed and with details on the model

variables not displayed, in order to provide a very basic overview of the obese cohort.

The normal-weight cohort model is identical in structure.

Figure 3.1: Obese Cohort, Subtrees Collapsed, Variables Hidden

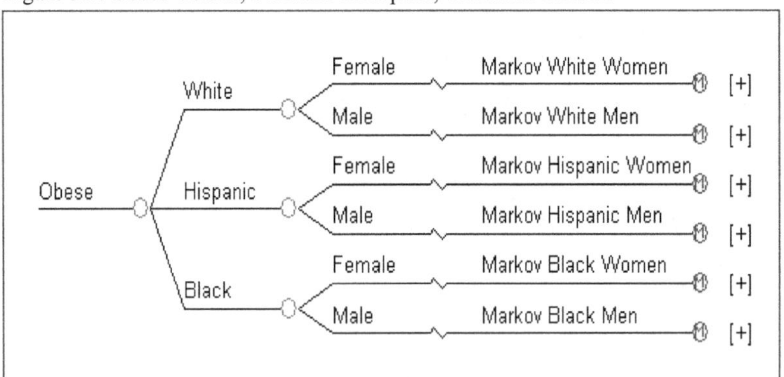

The methodology used here to calculate the external costs of obesity is based on that used by Tucker et al. (2006). Tucker et al.'s article estimated healthcare and quality of life costs for four hypothetical cohorts of overweight and obese 20 year olds. The approach of this dissertation differs from the Tucker et al. study however, as the Tucker analysis included other internal costs, e.g., costs related to quality of life, and did not include external costs associated with obesity, such as disability or pension payments. In addition, the Tucker study developed and reported on single race/sex 1000 person cohorts (e.g., black women, white men), whereas the cohorts detailed in the study described here are of mixed race/ethnicity and include both sexes.

The following sections describe the development of the model in detail. First, an introduction to key concepts in the Markov model is provided. The subsequent sub-sections describe in turn: cohort demographics; BMI; costs; probabilities; and discounting and interest rates. The final section provides an explanation of the cost calculation in TreeAge, and provides images of the model developed for the present study.

Markov Model: Key Concepts

A Markov model, also called a "state-transition" model, allows the iterative processing of a decision tree over a specified period. A *cycle* represents the time period it takes for the model to run once; *states* are mutually exclusive conditions or roles that a person may occupy during one cycle; each member of the cohort *transitions* at the end of every cycle to one of the states (note that this may be the same state in which they started);

probabilities are assigned to initial states, and to the likelihood of the different transition options (TreeAge Software Inc., 2008).

In the model developed for this dissertation, there are three states and an absorbing state for each member of the cohorts; they may be a *Worker, SSDI Disabled,* a *Retiree, or Dead.* The first three of these states provide transition options at the end of each cycle. *Dead* is an absorbing state. All members of the cohort are assigned to the Worker state initially, then transition to other states based on assigned probabilities described in the sub-sections that follow, and summarized in Table 3.11. Figure 3.2 provides another image of the model developed here, with the subgroup of non-Hispanic white women expanded. All of the other subgroups have identical sub-trees, but are collapsed here to aid understanding. Cycles are equivalent to years in this model, and the model runs for 65 cycles/years. In the middle-right of the figure are the four mutually exclusive states to which a cohort member may belong: *Worker, SSDI Disabled, Retiree, or Dead.* These states and their transitions are explained in turn below:

- *Worker:* All members of the cohort start in the Worker state. At the end of each cycle (one year), they *transition,* that is, they may continue working (return to the Worker state), become disabled (move to the SSDI Disabled state), retire (move to the Retiree state), or die (move to the Dead state). The probabilities of transitioning to the different states are detailed in the section on probabilities later in this chapter, are summarized in Table 3.11 and shown in Figure 3.4. All workers in this model retire at age 65.

- *SSDI Disabled:* This state refers to those members of the cohort who become permanently disabled, and receive social security disability insurance. The term "SSDI Disabled" is used to distinguish between other forms of disability, for which one may not receive benefits. At the end of each cycle, those who are in this category may reenter the workforce (move to the Worker state), remain SSDI Disabled (remain in the SSDI Disabled category), or die. Probabilities for transitioning to each of these outcomes are described in detail in the section on probabilities, are summarized in Table 3.11 and shown in Figure 3.4. In keeping with US government policy, those who start receiving SSDI benefits before retirement continue to receive SSDI benefits after reaching retirement age, and do not receive social security retirement payments (Social Security Administration [SSA], 2008).

- *Retiree:* Those members of the cohort who are retirees either remain retired or die at the end of each cycle. The probability of death is based on the Fontaine lifetables, described in detail in the section on probabilities later in this chapter.

- *Dead:* Dead is an absorbing state.

Figure 3.2: Obese Cohort - White Women Subgroup Expanded

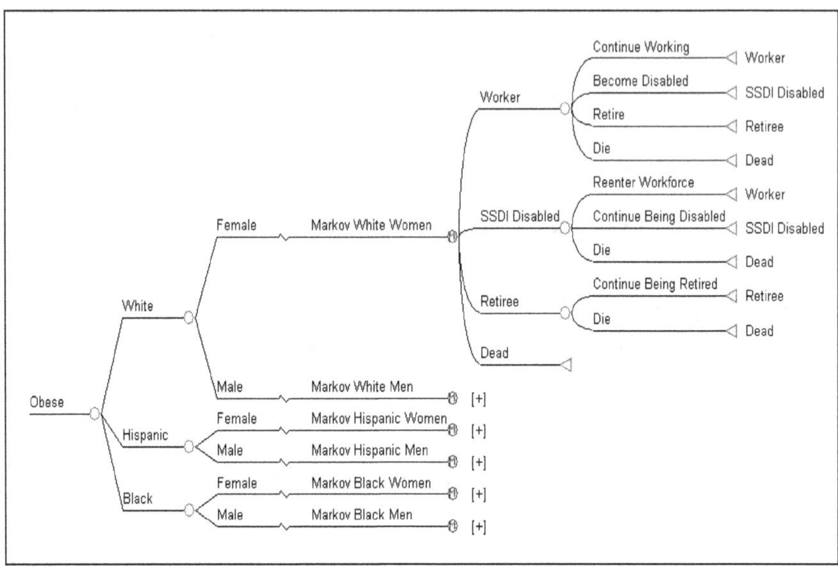

TreeAge allows costs for the different states and transition probabilities to be defined.

TreeAge then calculates total costs, given the assumptions of the model. The

assumptions, including costs and transition probabilities, are described in detail in the

Costs and Transition Probabilities sections and summarized in the Model Explanation

and Images section. Having reviewed some of the key concepts related to the model

developed here, the following section discusses the cohort demographics.

Cohort Demographics

The obese and normal weight 1000-person cohorts in the model developed here comprise

non-Hispanic whites, non-Hispanic blacks and Hispanics only, as national estimates of

obesity are provided only for these racial and ethnic groups (Ogden et al., 2006), and

together these racial and ethnic groups comprise 95% of the population in the US. Each obese and non-obese cohort is 70% non-Hispanic white, 16% Hispanic and 14% non-Hispanic black, reflecting the US population if it were limited to these three racial/ethnic groups. The demographic summary statistics of these racial and ethnic groups in the United States are provided in Table 3.1, in addition to percentage estimates of the US population for these groups if the population were limited to these groups only.

Table 3.1: U.S Population Summary Statistics

Race/Ethnicity	Population in US†	Percent of US Population Total†	Percent of US Population (If Limited to Hispanics, Non-Hispanic Blacks and Non-Hispanic Whites)
Non-Hispanic White	285.3 million	66%	69.786%
Non-Hispanic Black	40.7 million	13.5%	14.265%
Hispanic	45.5 million	15.1%	15.948%

†Source: US Census Bureau 2008

Men and women in the hypothetical cohorts account for 50% of each subgroup. The numbers of men and women in each racial/ethnic group in the obese and normal weight cohorts in the model are displayed in Table 3.2.

Table 3.2: Racial/Ethnic Makeup of Obese and Normal-Weight 1000-Person Cohorts

Race/Ethnicity	Percent of 1000 Person Cohort	Sex	Number in Cohort
Non-Hispanic White	70%	Men	350
		Women	350
Non-Hispanic Black	14%	Men	70
		Women	70
Hispanic	16%	Men	80
		Women	80

Having discussed cohort demographics, the next section provides an explanation of the treatment of BMI in the model.

BMI

This section provides an overview of the treatment of BMI in the model developed here

and discusses both *incremental BMI* and *starting BMIs* within the model. Other obesity-

related lifetime costing models employed different strategies to address BMI. Tucker et

al.'s study used starting BMIs of 30 for their obese cohorts and varied BMIs throughout

the cohort's lifetime. In Finkelstein et al. (2008), BMIs remained static throughout the

cohort's "lifetime". In the model developed for this dissertation, BMI varies over the

cohort's lifetime, and a range is used for starting BMIs of the obese cohort, in order to

better reflect obesity levels in the general U.S. population.

Incremental BMI

The BMI of a person tends to vary with age, however, not in a linear fashion. Instead,

BMI growth appears to be a function of age, sex, and initial BMI (Heo et al., 2003). Heo

et al. developed an algorithm that represents the BMI growth curve:

$$Y(t) = 0.266 + 0.0014\text{Age} - 0.036\text{Sex} + 0.985\text{BMI} + (0.759 - 0.0051\text{Age} -$$

$$0.026\text{Sex} - 0.016\text{BMI})t + (-0.0037 - 0.00011\text{Age} + 0.00033\text{Sex} + 0.00016\text{BMI})t^2$$

In this equation, *Age* is the age at baseline, *BMI* is the BMI at baseline, and *Sex* is 1 for

men and 0 for women, and *t* is the number of years from baseline. The model developed

for this dissertation uses this Heo et al. equation to modify BMI for the members of the

obese and normal weight cohorts based on starting BMI, age and sex.

Starting BMI

The starting BMI for the normal weight cohort in the model described here is 20. For the obese cohort, the starting BMI is a range of levels that varies by the race/ethnicity and sex of each sub-cohort, based on the best available population-level data. There is no data available specifically for obese 20-year olds in the United States, therefore the starting BMI was determined by using 1) figures of obesity BMI in children and adolescents, and 2) 20-39 year-old adults. Table 3.3 displays obesity prevalence in 20-39 year olds in the US by race and gender and levels of obesity.

Table 3.3: 2003-2004 US Population Obesity Prevalence by Sex, Race/Ethnicity in 20-39 year olds

Sex	Race/Ethnicity	(A) Percent of Population who is Obese (Obesity Classes I, II, III)	(B) Percent of Population who is Extremely Obese (Obesity Class III)	(B/A) Percentage of Obese who are Extremely Obesity
Males	Non-Hispanic white	27.2	3.2	11.76
	Non-Hispanic Black	32.3	7.1	21.98
	Mexican American	32.7	1.9	5.81
Females	Non-Hispanic white	23.8	6.4	26.89
	Non-Hispanic Black	50.3	15.7	31.21
	Mexican American	35.7	8.6	24.08

Source: Ogden et al., 2006

The starting range of numbers in each obesity category for each of the six race/ethnicity and gender-based sub-cohorts is displayed in Table 3.4. Nationally representative figures on obesity for **children and adolescents 2-19**, and **adults 20-39** are used to calculate the starting BMI ranges for the 20-year old cohort. Briefly, the obesity class III figures reflect the percentage of **children and adolescents 2-19** who are morbidly obese. The obesity

class II percentages of the cohort, when summed with the obesity class III percentages

equal the percentages of **adults 20-39** who are morbidly obese (obesity class III),

according to the most recent NHANES figures, shown in Table 3.3 . The starting obesity

class I figures are equal to the total persons in the subgroup, minus obesity classes II and

III. This calculation of the figures for each obesity category by race/ethnicity and gender

is described in greater detail below. The sub-group starting distributions are summarized

in the "StartDist" table variables (which differ by race/ethnicity and gender) provided in

Appendix B.

Table 3.4: Makeup of Hypothetical Cohort of Obese 1000-person Cohort at Age 20 by
Race/Ethnicity and Starting BMI

Race/Ethnicity	Sex	BMI 30 (Obesity Class I)	BMI 39 (Obesity Class II)	BMI 40 (Obesity Class III)	Total Persons
Non-Hispanic white (70%)	Men	309	25	16	350
	Women	256	84	10	350
Non-Hispanic Black (14%)	Men	55	12	3	70
	Women	48	20	2	70
Hispanic (16%)	Men	75	1	4	80
	Women	61	17	2	80
Total		**804**	**159**	**37**	**1000**

Column 1 (the percentage for each race/ethnicity) is sourced from column 4 in Table 3.2.

Column 6 (total persons) represents the total number of persons in a 1000 person cohort,

based on the percentage in Column 1, and assumes the number of men and women in

each race/ethnicity are divided equally. *Column 5* (obesity class III) is the number of each

sub-cohort who is morbidly obese at age 20. According to a forthcoming study of

NHANES data (Wang, personal communication, 17th October, 2008), 4.6% of boys and 2.9% of girls 2-19 in the US are morbidly obese. Therefore, for the purposes of this model, 4.6% of men and 2.9% of women of each sub-group in the obese cohort are also morbidly obese (obesity class III) initially, although this may underestimate the actual numbers of morbidly obese in for each sub-cohort. Column 5 represents 4.6% or 2.9% of the total in Column 6 for men and women respectively, rounded to the nearest whole number.

Column 4 (obesity class II) represents those who would have a BMI of around 40 by age 40, using the Heo et al. algorithm described above, minus of the number already classed as morbidly obese at age 20 (Column 5). *Column 3* (BMI 30) in Table 3.4 is the total number of persons in the sub-cohort, minus the number of persons in Columns 4 and 5. The next section discusses the cost inputs to the model.

Costs

Having reviewed the model's basic structure, cohort demographics and treatment of BMI both at start and throughout the course of the model, this section provides an overview of the cost inputs to the model and the derivation of those costs. Table 3.5 provides an overview of the costing areas relevant to obesity located by the costing literature meta-analysis and literature review in Chapter Two, and notes whether these represent "internal" or "external" costs. If a cost is internal, it is borne by the individual; if it is external, it is borne by society. Only external costs are used in the calculation of the model for this dissertation. The cost inputs to the model discussed in this section include:

absenteeism, social security disability insurance, productivity, social security retirement benefits, and wages/tax foregone. All of the costs described here are operationalized as variables in the TreeAge model developed for this dissertation. Details on these variables are provided in Appendix A. The names of the variables that are related to costing start with a lower-case "c".

Table 3.5: Summary of Lifetime Costs Impacted by Obesity

Type of Cost	**Internal Cost**	**External Cost**
Quality of life	Quality of life	
Absenteeism		Sick leave payments
Disability insurance		Disability payments
Healthcare	Healthcare out of pocket expenses	Balance of healthcare costs
Productivity		Productivity
Retirement		Social Security payments
Wages/tax revenue	Wages	Tax revenue

Absenteeism

Table 3.6 displays the costing inputs for absenteeism (short-term absence from work) used in the model developed for this dissertation. These cost estimates derive from Finkelstein et al. (2005b). This was the only study located in the obesity costing meta-analysis, shown in Table 4.2 that 1) measured the cost of absenteeism using three levels of obesity, and 2) used nationally representative data in its analysis. The Finkelstein study's results report lower than expected costs for the severely obese for both men and women. This may reflect sampling issues of the severely obese working population in the study itself. However, it suggests also that the costing estimates used in the model developed here may be conservative.

Table 3.6: Absenteeism Costing Inputs

Gender	BMI	Original Costs Above Normal Weight ($2004)	$2007 Costs (Model Input)
Men	30-34.9	$ 70	$ 76.83
	35-39.9	$643	$ 705.78
	40+	$436	$ 478.57
Women	30-34.9	$302	$ 331.48
	35-39.9	$936	$1,027.38
	40+	$805	$ 883.59

Source for Original Costs: Finkelstein et al. 2005b

Social Security Disability Insurance

Workers who become totally disabled and unable to work are eligible for Social Security

Disability Insurance benefits (Social Security Administration [SSA], 2008b). Note that

the Social Security Administration (SSA) definition of disability does not include short-

term disability or partial disability (SSA, 2008b). Table 3.7 displays a summary of the

disability insurance benefits used in the model developed for this dissertation, by age and

gender. The probability that one will receive disability insurance benefits is discussed in

the section that follows on probabilities.

Table 3.7: Average Monthly and Annual Disability Insurance Benefit Payments by Sex and Age, 2007

Gender	Age Range	Monthly Average Benefit ($2007)‡	Annual Average Benefit ($2007) (Model Input)
Men	Under 25	$549.10	$6,589.20
	25 - 29	$669.10	$8,029.20
	30 - 34	$763.10	$9,157.20
	35 - 39	$845.60	$10,147.20
	40 - 44	$917.20	$11,006.40
	45 - 49	$1,004.70	$12,056.40
	50 - 54	$1,111.90	$13,342.80
	55 - 59	$1,226.30	$14,715.60
	60 - 64	$1,312.40	$15,748.80
Women	Under 25	$519.90	$6,238.80
	25 - 29	$636.60	$7,639.20
	30 - 34	$720.20	$8,642.40
	35 - 39	$781.60	$9,379.20
	40 - 44	$821.40	$9,856.80
	45 - 49	$853.90	$10,246.80
	50 - 54	$887.00	$10,644.00
	55 - 59	$911.10	$10,933.20
	60 - 64	$898.20	$10,778.40

‡Source: (Social Security Administration, 2008a)

Healthcare

Table 3.8 contains a summary of the healthcare-related costing inputs for the model.

These costs were sourced from two studies estimating the healthcare costs associated

with obesity: Finkelstein, Fiebelkorn and Wang (2005b) and Andreyeva, Sturm, and

Ringel (2004). These studies are included in the summary of healthcare costing in Table

4.1. The studies were chosen as inputs for the model based on: whether the study sample

was representative of the US population, the age range of the study sample, the

granularity of the obesity levels in the study (i.e., whether there were the study delineated

between the multiple levels of obesity), and how recently the study was performed.

Two studies were used as sources for the model healthcare costing inputs for ages 20-85, as no single study provided costing information that was both representative of the US population and for three levels of obesity. The age range under study for the Finkelstein article was 18-64. In the model developed here, Finkelstein's figures are used for ages 20-65, and Andreyeva's figures are used for ages 65-85, even though the age range for the Andreyeva study was 54-69. The higher age in the Andreyeva range is not substantially greater than for the Finkelstein study. However, no study was located that assessed healthcare costs for US adults 65-85 and that used nationally representative data, and assessed costs for all three levels of obesity. Medical costs tend to increase with age, and this at least is reflected in the Andreyeva study. It is also likely that the costing inputs for the ages 65-85 in the model derived from the Andreyeva study are conservative, given the age range of the study is 54-69.

Table 3.8 displays the healthcare costs included in the model developed here for obese persons over those for normal weight, by sex, age range, and obesity level, by dollar/year, as calculated by the authors of the original studies. In the final column, these costs are translated into 2007 dollars, using the Medical Consumer Price Index (MCPI). The final column of Table 3.8 shows 75.8% of the total 2007 costs. According to the Centers for Medicare and Medicaid Services (CMS), healthcare costs borne by individuals represented 24.2% of total healthcare spending in the US in 2007 (Centers for Medicare and Medicaid Services [CMS], nd). These individual costs included (1) out-of-pocket spending, such as deductibles and co-pays, and (2) private insurance, which includes private spending on insurance premiums. Out-of pocket spending represented 12.2% of national healthcare spending in 2007; private insurance: 12% (CMS, nd). In the analysis

presented here, we are only interested in calculating external costs, so 75.8% (100 -

24.2%) of healthcare costs will be used as inputs to the model.

Table 3.8: Healthcare Costing Inputs

Gender	Age	BMI	Original Costs: Greater than Normal Weight (Year)‡	$2007 Costs	$2007 Costs *.758
Men	Ages 20-65	30-34-9	$ 392 ($2004)	$ 444.77	$ 337.14
		35-39.9	$ 569 ($2004)	$ 645.60	$ 489.37
		40+	$1,591 ($2004)	$1,805.19	$1,368.33
	Ages 65+	30-34-9	$ 823 ($2002)	$1,015.83	$ 770.00
		35-39.9	$2,264 ($2002)	$2,794.46	$2,118.20
		40+	$4,102 ($2002)	$5,063.11	$3,837.84
Women	Ages 20-65	30-34-9	$1,071 ($2004)	$1,220.86	$ 925.41
		35-39.9	$1,549 ($2004)	$1,757.54	$1,332.22
		40+	$1,359 ($2004)	$1,541.96	$1,168.81
	Ages 65+	30-34-9	$1,094 ($2002)	$1,350.33	$1,023.55
		35-39.9	$1,732 ($2002)	$2,137.81	$1,620.46
		40+	$4,449 ($2002)	$5,491.41	$4,162.49

‡ Source: Finkelstein et al., 2005b; Andreyeva et al., 2004

Productivity

"Productivity" in this dissertation signifies the reduced output of a worker. The

productivity costing information for the lifetime costing model is provided in Table 3.9.

Only one study (Ricci & Chee, 2005) located by the costing literature costing analysis

(summarized in Table 4.4) used nationally representative data in assessing costs of

productivity. The results of the study are limited to one overall category of obesity: BMI

of 30+. The costs are converted from the original costs reported in the study to $2007

costs using the CPI index.

Table 3.9: Productivity Costing Inputs

Gender	BMI	Original Annual Costs Greater than Normal Weight ($2002)‡	$2007 Costs
Men & Women	30+	$1,090	$1,256.27

‡ Source: Ricci & Chee, 2005

Social Security Retirement Benefits

As discussed in Chapter One and in the study by Fontaine et al. (2003), BMI impacts

mortality rates. Earlier mortality will, in turn, reduce total social security retirement

benefits collected over a person's lifetime. Therefore, it is important to include retirement

benefits when estimating lifetime costs of obesity. According to the Social Security

Administration (SSA), the average monthly benefit for retired workers in May, 2008 was

$1083.60 (SSA, 2008c). Thus, the yearly figure for retirement benefits would be

$13,003.20. This amount would be equivalent to $12,445.70 in 2007 dollars. In the

model described here, all workers who are alive and not SSDI disabled, retire at age 65

and start receiving retirement benefits. Current full retirement age in the United States is

67 years, however recipients are eligible to start receiving benefits at a reduced rate after

age 62 (SSA, 2008d). The model described here uses average annual retirement benefits

as costs, therefore, 65 was chosen as the retirement age as it is the nearest whole number

average of 62 and 67.

Wages (Tax Foregone)

As noted in Chapter Two, several studies have shown that there is a persistent wage

effect of obesity, although the causal mechanism for this disparity is debated (Pagan &

Davlia, 1997; Averett & Korenman, 1996; Baum & Ford, 2004; Bhattacharya & Bundorf,

2005). Calculation of tax foregone is not mentioned specifically in the obesity costing literature. However, it would appear prudent to include this cost in the calculations. Therefore, for the purposes of the model developed here, an annual cost of $324 per obese worker is used. This figure is derived from the following: The median annual wage in 2007 was $40,690 (Bureau of Labor Statistics [BLS], 2007) and Baum and Ford (2004) found that for obese workers, wages decreased relative to workers of normal weight in the range 0.7 to 6.3%. Assuming the average of Baum and Ford's range (3.185%), median wages would be lowered to $39,394 given this wage effect. Tax rates in 2007 for this salary range were $4,386.25 plus 25% of the amount over $31,850 (Internal Revenue Service [IRS], 2007). Federal tax on $40,690 would therefore be $6,596.25, and tax on $39,394 would be $6,272.25, a difference of $324. As state taxes vary so widely throughout the US, and are likely to be much smaller than federal taxes, state tax calculations have not been included in the model developed here.

Transition Probabilities

Having examined the major costing inputs to the model, we now turn to a discussion of the transition probabilities. Some of the transition probabilities described here are operationalized as variables in the TreeAge model. Transition probabilities are defined in TreeAge for each transition option, often using Boolean logic. Details on the transition probability variables are provided in Appendix A, and start with a lower-case "p". Greater detail is provided on important probabilities in the sections that follow, including probability of death, the probability of becoming SSDI disabled, and probability of returning to work once SSDI disabled.

Probability of Death

The study detailed here utilizes life tables developed in a 2003 study by Fontaine et al., which examined the effect of BMI levels on mortality. To develop lifetables that estimated the effect of BMI, age, gender and race/ethnicity on mortality, Fontaine and colleagues drew from the US life tables (1999), the third annual NHANES survey (1988-1994), the First National Health and Nutrition Epidemiologic Follow up Study (NHANES I and II) and NHANES II Mortality Study (1976-1992). The results from their research were published in the *Journal of the American Medical Association*, and the tables are available online:

http://www.soph.uab.edu/statgenetics/Research/Tables/YLL.htm). These Fontaine et al.-developed lifetables were transcribed into Excel v7.0 format (Microsoft corporation, Redmond Washington), and then loaded as tables into TreeAge. These transcribed lifetables are also provided in Appendix C.

The Fontaine et al. tables generally show a J or U shaped risk of mortality associated with BMI levels. For example, it is estimated that 20 year-old white men with BMI levels of 25, 30, 35, 40 and 45 would lose 0, 1, 3, 6 and 13 years of life respectively, and 50-year-old white men would lose 0, 0, 3, 4 and 7 years of life respectively. The association between BMI and mortality differed between genders and between racial groups. The association for 20-year-olds between BMI levels, age, gender and race/ethnicity, is shown in Figure 3.3. For example, a 20-year old black man with a BMI of 45 would expect to lose 20 years of life on average. It appears however, that overweight and lower levels of obesity may in fact be protective for black women. This anomaly is not fully explained in the Fontaine et al. article, although it may be due to confounding effects in the study

sample used to determine life expectancy estimates.

Figure 3.3: Estimated Years of Life Lost at Age 20 Years by BMI Level, Race/Ethnicity
and Gender

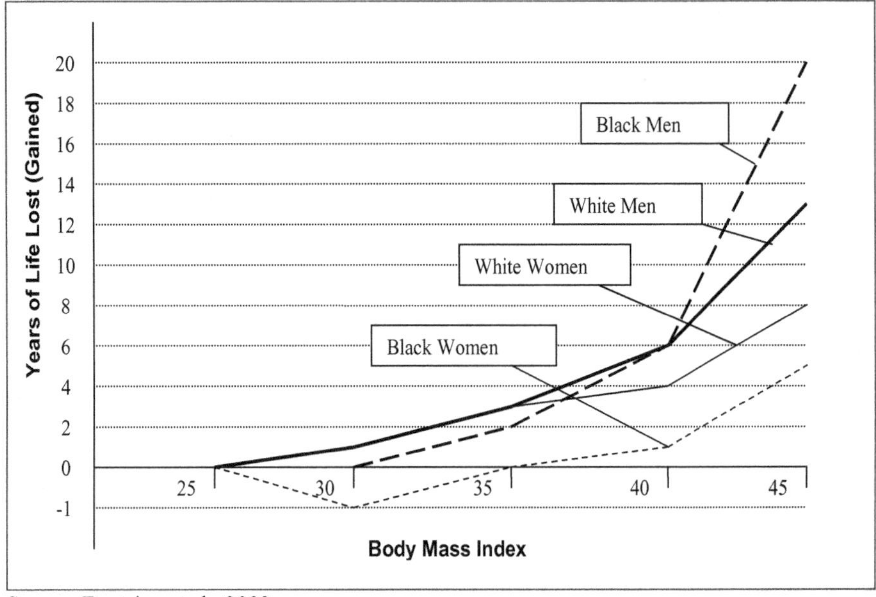

Source: Fontaine et al., 2003

Social Security Disability Insurance

Table 3.10 displays the number of workers in the United States in 2007 and the

beneficiaries of social security disability insurance, by age and gender. The probability

that one will be disabled is calculated by dividing the number of workers receiving SSDI

benefits, by the sum of those beneficiaries and the total number of workers in the US.

This represents the "baseline" probability of receiving disability insurance for the

workers in the United States.

Table 3.10: US Employment and Disability Figures 2007

Gender	Age Range	Number of Workers (A)‡	Workers Receiving SSDI Benefits (B)†	Percentage of Workers Receiving SSDI Benefits (C) 100*[B/(A+B)]	Disability Probability (Percentage of Workers Receiving Benefits / Number of Years in Age Range) (C/5)
Men	Under 25	10,291,000	29,003	0.28%	0.056%
	25 - 29	8,943,000	86,530	0.95%	0.19%
	30 - 34	8,509,000	118,519	1.37%	0.274%
	35 - 39	9,221,000	192,012	2.04%	0.408%
	40 - 44	9,445,000	314,743	3.22%	0.644%
	45 - 49	9,677,000	483,943	4.76%	0.952%
	50 - 54	8,533,000	643,244	7.01%	1.402%
	55 - 59	6,628,000	825,507	11.08%	2.216%
	60 - 64	3,927,000	932,822	19.19%	3.383%
Women	Under 25	9,584,000	19,988	0.21%	0.042%
	25 - 29	7,304,000	69,937	0.95%	0.19%
	30 - 34	6,829,000	111,023	1.6%	0.32%
	35 - 39	7,456,000	181,609	2.38%	0.476%
	40 - 44	8,180,000	288,752	3.41%	0.682%
	45 - 49	8,608,000	437,617	4.84%	0.968%
	50 - 54	7,745,000	584,975	7.02%	1.404%
	55 - 59	6,063,000	725,575	10.69%	2.138%
	60 - 64	3,489,000	784,345	18.35%	3.67%

Source: ‡BLS, 2008; †SSA, 2008a

According to the results of the disability costing literature, summarized in Table 4.3, estimates of the impact of obesity on the likelihood of receiving a disability pension in Scandinavian countries (where most of this research has taken place) ranges from 35% increased risk for those with BMI $\geq$30 (Karnehed, Rassmussen & Kark, 2007) to over 300% for those of BMI $\geq$35 (Neovius, Kark, & Rasmussen, 2008). Given the increased risk of disease caused by obesity, and the strong linkage between obesity and disability pension payments reported in Scandinavian countries, it seems reasonable to conclude that obesity levels in the United States would also influence the likelihood of receiving SSDI benefits. However, given that there has been little work on this estimated impact in the US, and the likelihood of the Scandinavian benefits being more generous than in the US (which may act as a greater incentive to apply to receive disability insurance), these impacts have been estimated conservatively at baseline at a 10% increased risk for persons whose BMI is 30-34.9 and 30% increased risk for people whose BMIs are $\geq$35. A sensitivity analysis on these assumptions is performed and reported on in Chapter Four. The association between obesity and disability insurance in the US may be a fruitful topic for future research.

Probability of Returning to Work Once Receiving Disability Insurance

The Social Security Administration (2008a) reports that 33,381 persons returned to work in 2007 after receiving social security disability insurance benefits from a total of 7,098,723 beneficiaries. Dividing 33,381 by 7,098,723 is 0.0047. Therefore, in the model developed here, the probability of returning to work once receiving SSDI benefits is 0.0047.

Discounting and Interest Rates

Having discussed both the costs and probabilities that are used as inputs to the model developed for this dissertation, this section reviews other another key set of assumptions: discounting and interest rates. The rates described here are operationalized as variables in the TreeAge model. Details on these variables are provided in Appendix A. The names of the variables that are related to rates start with "Rate_". The rates below describe the assumptions in the baseline model. However, these baseline rates are varied in a later sensitivity analysis, the results of which are described in Chapter Four.

Discounting

Due to the effects of inflation, future expenses or savings will be worth less than expenses or savings in today's dollars, therefore it is important to discount these future costs. A discount rate of 5% is used, as is standard in most government cost-benefit analyses.

Interest Rate

According to the Bureau of Labor Statistics, average annual Consumer Price Index CPI and Medical CPI increases from 2000 to 2007 (inclusive) were respectively 2.8% and 4.3% (BLS, 2008b). The model developed for this dissertation uses these average increases as inputs at 2.8% for non-medical costs, and 4.3% for healthcare costs for its baseline calculations.

Model Explanation and Images

After describing inputs to the model, such as costing, transition probabilities and rates, this section provides a short explanation of the model's calculations, as well as images of the model developed here in TreeAge Pro 2009.

Figure 3.4: Obese Cohort, White Women Sub-group: Costs and Transition Probabilities Displayed

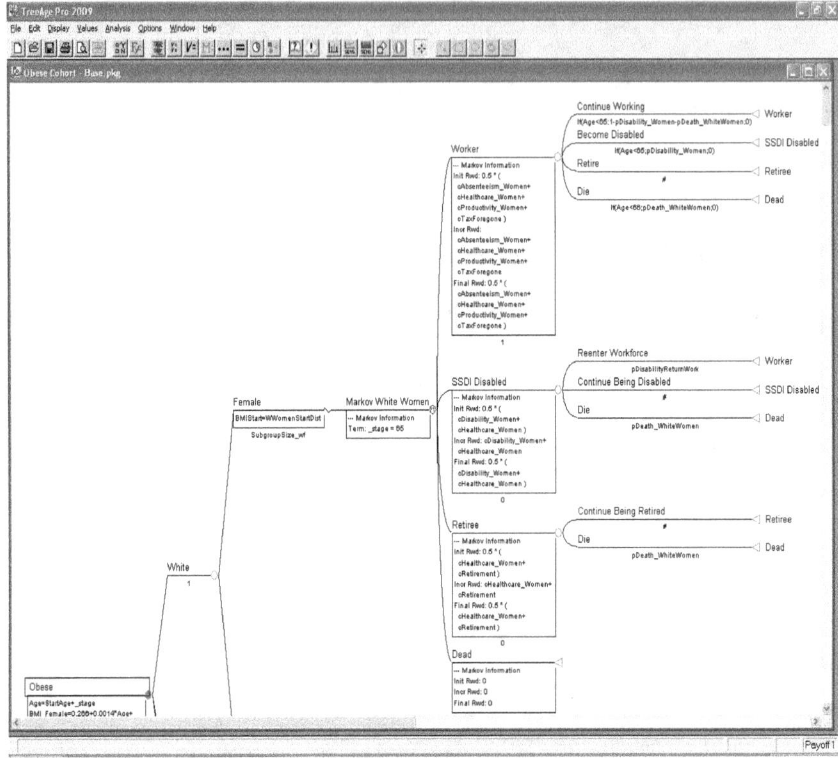

Figure 3.4 shows a screen shot of the non-Hispanic white women sub-cohort with costing

information and transition probabilities displayed. All other gender and racial/ethnic

subgroups are identical in structure, but may differ in some of the costs and variables

used. In order for TreeAge to calculate the lifetime costs of the cohort, both costs and

transition probabilities are defined in the software. Once all of these costs and transition

probabilities and any other variables are defined, a feature in TreeAge —"rollback"—

calculates the total costs given the specified model assumptions. The subsections below

summarize the costing and transition probabilities for the model developed in the present

study.

Model Costing

Costs were entered for each state (Worker, SSDI Disabled or Retiree) under each of those

states in the TreeAge software. For example, a Worker in the obese cohort incurs greater

costs than the normal weight cohort in the following areas: healthcare, absenteeism, taxes

foregone and reduced productivity. These costs may be seen under the Worker state in

Figure 3.4. Table 3.11 displays a summary of the costing inputs by state, as defined in

the TreeAge model developed for this dissertation. The costs section earlier in this

chapter details the how each of the costs were derived. Please note that actual variable

names in the model differ by gender. Details on each of the costing variables are provided

in Appendix A, and start with a lower-case "c".

Table 3.11: Costing Variables Defined for Each Cycle, by State ($2007)

State	**Costing Variables Defined for each Cycle, by State**	**Source for Costing / Explanation**
Worker	cHealthcare_*Gender*†	Table 3.8
	cAbsenteeism_ *Gender*†	Table 3.6
	cProductivity_ *Gender*†	Table 3.9
	cTaxForegone	$ 345
SSDI Disabled	cHealthcare_ *Gender*†	Table 3.8
	cDisability_ *Gender*†	Table 3.7
Retiree	cHealthcare_ *Gender*†	Table 3.8
	cRetirement	$12,445.70

† Men or Women

Model Transition Options and Probabilities

In addition to the costing information, transition options and probabilities must be

defined. In Figure 3.4, the transition options and probabilities are displayed to the right of

each of the states. For example, at the end of each year, a Worker may: continue

working, become disabled, retire, or die. The derivation of each of the probabilities for

these options is discussed in the previous section in this chapter on transition probabilities. The transition probabilities are entered in the TreeAge software underneath

the option itself, as shown in Figure 3.4. Table 3.12 provides a summary of the

definitions of all of the transition probabilities in the model developed for the present

study by state, and their derivation. Each of the transition probability variables begin with

a lowercase "p", and are explained in detail in Appendix A.

Table 3.12: Transition Options and Probabilities by Markov Model State

State	Transition Option	Probability Expression Defined in the TreeAge Model	Comment/Explanation
Worker	Continue Working	If (Age<65; 1 - pDisability_*Gender*† - pDeath_*Race/Ethn*‡*Gender*†; 0)	If under 65, all who do not become SSDI Disabled or die, continue working
	Become SSDI Disabled	If (Age<65; pDisability_*Gender*†;0)	If under 65, transition to the SSDI Disabled state based on the pDisability Tables in Appendix B, derived from the information in Table 3.11
	Retire	#	All workers who have not become SSDI Disabled and have not died, retire at age 65. The # symbol in TreeAge is an "automatic probability complement" calculator, i.e., it signifies the remainder of all other probabilities
	Die	If (Age<66; pDeath_*Race/Ethn*‡*Gender*†; 0)	If 65 or under, use the appropriate race and gender probability tables created by Fontaine et al. (2003) to calculate probability of death by age and BMI. The probability of death tables are shown in Appendix C
SSDI Disabled	Return to Work	pDisabilityReturnWork	Return to work, based on the probability calculated in the subsection on SSDI Disability Insurance: 0.0047
	Continue Being SSDI Disabled	#	All those who are SSDI Disabled who do not return to work or die, remain SSDI Disabled. SSDI benefits become retirement benefits after reaching the qualifying age (SSA, 2008a)
	Die	pDisability_*Gender*†	Use the appropriate race and gender probability tables created by Fontaine et al. (2003) to calculate probability of death by age and BMI
Retire	Continue Being Retired	#	All those Retirees who do not die, remain Retired
	Die	pDisability_*Gender*†	Use the appropriate race and gender probability tables created by Fontaine et al. (2003) to calculate probability of death by age and BMI

† Men or Women

‡ Black, White, or Hispanic

This sub-section displays other images of the model developed for this dissertation, which is challenging given the size of the model developed for the present study. If printed out in 14 point font, and with all details displayed, the model is approximately 40 inches high by 22 inches wide. Please note that *all* of the images provided in this chapter (Figures 3.1-3.2 and 3.4-3.7) display the same model and vary only in terms of different subtrees that are collapsed or expanded, variables and Markov details that are displayed or hidden. Figure 3.5 shows the model with all the variables displayed, but with the sub-groups collapsed. These variables and their definitions are also described in detail in Appendix A. Figure 3.6 shows the model of the obese cohort with the subgroups expanded, but variables hidden. Figure 3.7 shows the entire model with subgroups and variables. While not legible, the image may aid conceptual understanding.

Figure 3.5: Obese Cohort: Variables Displayed, Sub-groups Collapsed

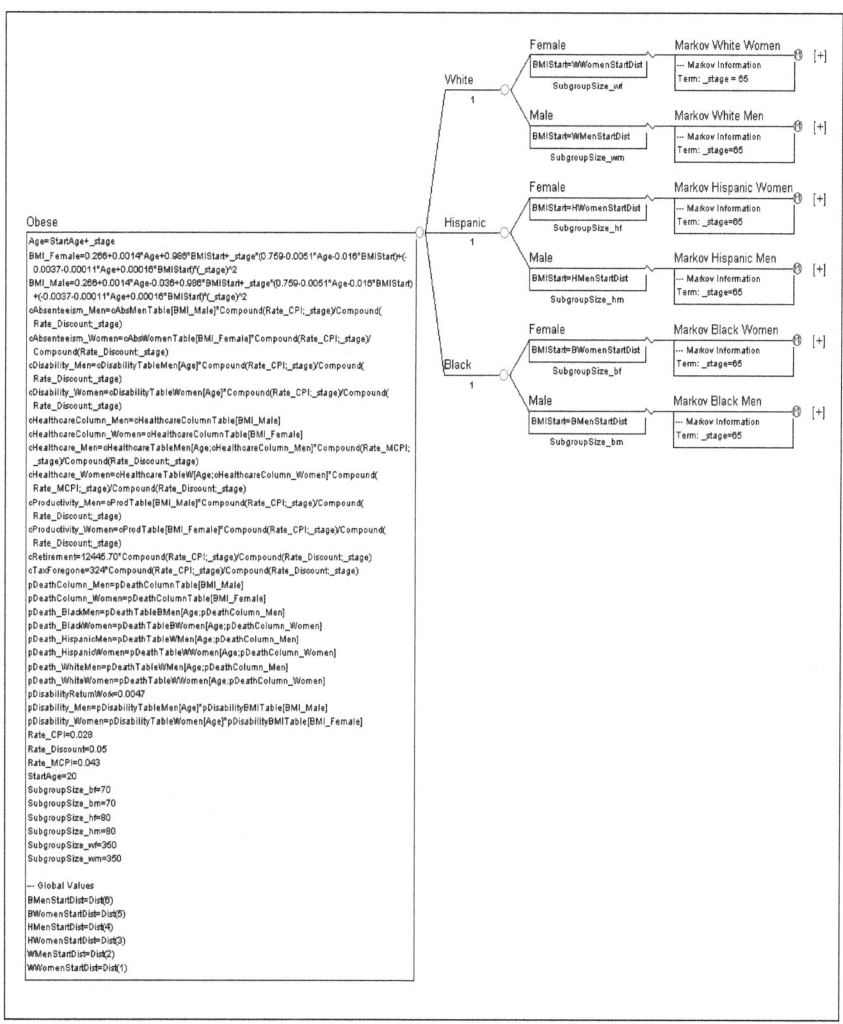

Figure 3.6: Obese

Cohort, Subgroups

Expanded, Variables

Hidden

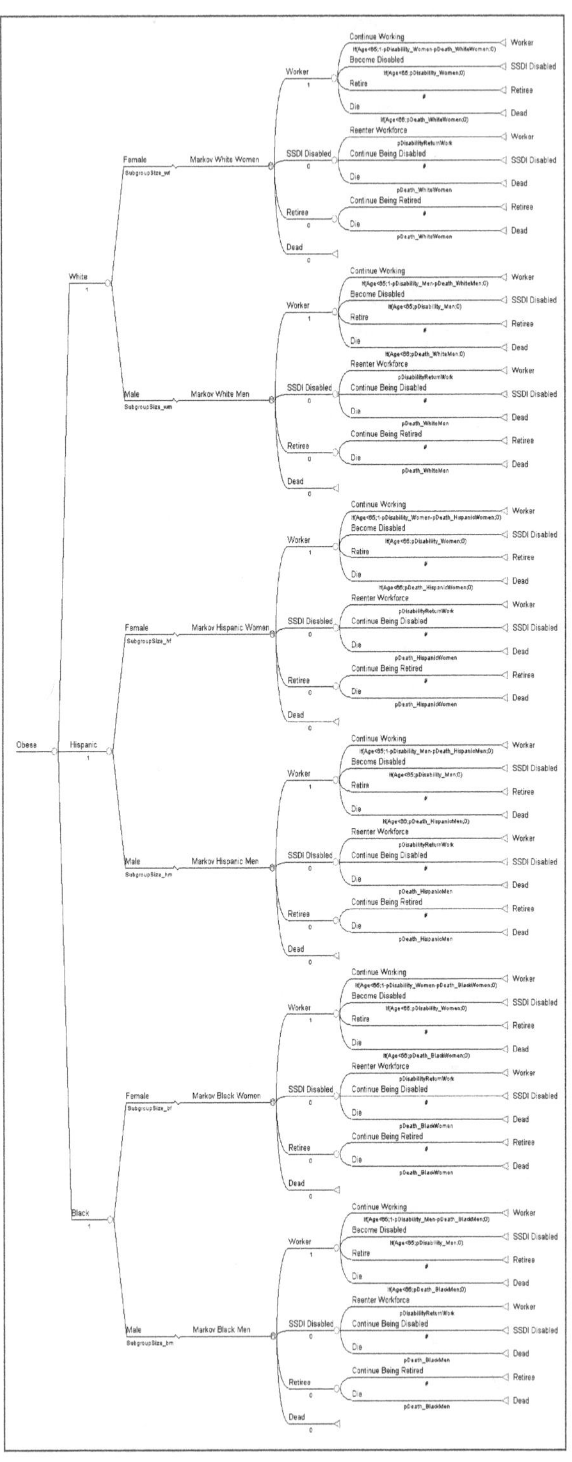

Figure 3.7: Obese Cohort:

Subgroups Expanded, Variables

Displayed

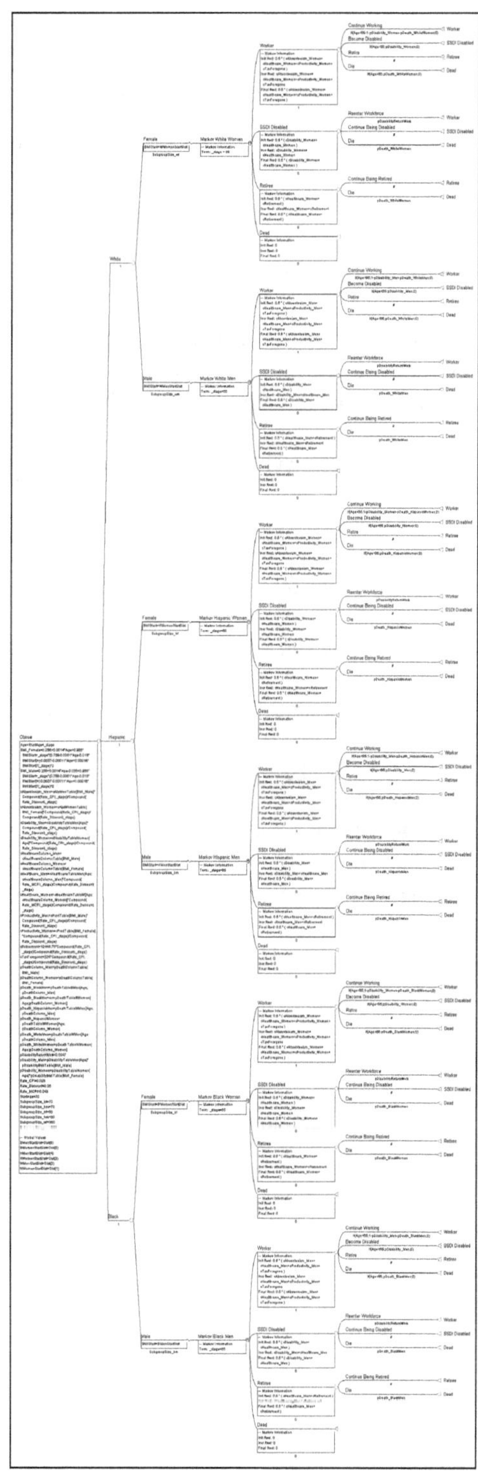

Conclusion

This chapter detailed the methodology of the analysis undertaken for this dissertation. The methodology has two phases. Phase One is a meta-analysis if the existing costing literature related to obesity. Phase Two uses the results from the first phase to identify many of the external costs associated with obesity. In Phase Two, a Markov model is developed using simulation software to calculate and compare the net present value of the lifetime, external costs of 20-year-old, 1000-person obese and normal weight cohorts that are racially/ethnically similar to the current United States population.

The author acknowledges that the model described here is not a perfect representation of the US population and their life progression; not all adults are employed at age 20, work continuously throughout their lives, and retire at 65, for example. However, best efforts were made by the author on the inputs to the model and its representativeness. In addition, the **comparative costs**—given the same assumptions—between the obese and normal weight cohorts are of greatest interest in this analysis. The following chapter reports on the results of the analysis described here.

Chapter Four: Results

Introduction

This chapter presents the findings of the study described here. The chapter (1) reviews and synthesizes the costing studies related to obesity published in the peer-reviewed literature between January 1990 and July 2008, and (2) reports on the results of the Markov model, which estimates the net present value of the lifetime, external costs of obesity. The results of the literature meta-analysis show that obesity-related costing studies fall into the following five categories: healthcare, absenteeism, disability insurance, productivity and other. Collectively, these studies show a strong association between obesity and costs, and the association generally increases with higher BMI levels. This review also informs the lifetime costing model in Phase Two by determining several of the model categories and inputs. Results from the Markov model suggest that increased rates of obesity in the United States result in substantial financial externalities.

Phase One Results

Over 100 studies were located using the search criteria described in Chapter Three and were reviewed by the author. Of these studies, 56 met the inclusion criteria and in are included the summary tables presented here. The 56 studies may be divided into five main categories: healthcare, absenteeism, productivity, disability and other. These categories are discussed in turn in the following sections.

There are five important points regarding the summary of the costing literature presented here:

1) Several of the located studies assessed costs in more than one category. Therefore, the same study may be appear in more than one of the following sections, but only information relevant to that costing area is provided in the study summary.

2) The language used to describe costing areas is often inconsistent between studies. Researchers often use the term "productivity" as a general phrase to signify the overall contribution by workers and is commonly used to include absenteeism, disability and reduced performance while at work (e.g., Burton, Chen, Schutz, & Edington,1999). In this dissertation, "productivity" is used to denote decreased performance at work only.

   Another example of language inconsistency between studies was the use of the term "disability". For some, the term was used to denote work-related short-term disability (less than six months), for others it meant work-related long-term disability (six months or greater). For others still, disability referred to the impaired ability to complete activities of daily living, which may or may not be related to employment. However, when estimating costs associated with obesity, most researchers appeared to associate short-term disability with absenteeism. Long-term disability on the other hand was generally used to denote extended absence from work that may be permanent, and was equated with disability insurance. In this dissertation, the term "absenteeism" is used to denote illness-related short-term absence from work, and includes costs associated both with

absenteeism and short-term disability. "Disability" is used to denote the category

of studies assessing costs related to social security disability insurance, also called

disability retirement or disability pension in other countries.

3) Many researchers, but not all, explicitly include the dollar/year information for

which their studies assessed costs. If the researcher provided dollar/year

information in their published study, it was included in the summary information

in the summary tables at the top of the findings section and in bold. If the

information was not available, it was not included in the summary tables.

4) BMI cutoffs used to denote normal weight, overweight and levels of obesity were

not standard across the studies included in the meta-analysis, and these differing

cutoffs are noted in the summary tables. For many studies from the early 1990s,

BMI of approximately 27 was used to distinguish between overweight and

obesity. Later in the 1990s, most studies appear to adopt the standards that are

provided in the front section of this dissertation, with BMIs of 18.5, 25, and 30 as

the common cut-off points. Relatively few of the located studies differentiated

between categories I, II and III of obesity, which equate to BMIs of 30-34.9, 35-

39.9 and 40+ respectively. However, the studies that did make this differentiation

in obesity level often show substantial differences in costs between these obesity

categories. It is also important to note that some studies group underweight and

normal weight individuals together by classifying a BMI of less than 25 as "normal". This may impact their findings, as many who are underweight are so because of the result of illness.

5) Finally, relatively few of the studies used nationally representative data in estimating costs, often analyzing convenience sample data. Thus, while the results of these studies may be helpful in the context of the study sector/population, they are not representative of the US population, and were not used as inputs to the costing model developed for this dissertation. The sections below describe and summarize the results of the meta-analysis of the costing studies, which fall into the categories of: healthcare, absenteeism, disability, productivity and "other".

Healthcare Costing

A total of 35 articles were located that calculated healthcare costs associated with obesity in the United States from January 1990 to December 2008. These studies are summarized in Table 4.1. Overall, the studies show a strong, positive correlation between increasing weight and healthcare costs. The approaches taken by researchers to analyze these costs differ by: unit of analysis, such as by individual or the economy as a whole; methodology; sample population and temporal period, which are described in more detail in the following sub-sections.

Unit of Analysis

Costs assessed at the individual level show increased healthcare costs for obese persons. However, these costs vary according to the breakdown in obesity levels used in the study.

If greater granularity was provided, results generally show a 'J-shaped' relationship between BMI level and healthcare costs, with substantially higher costs for obesity categories II and III (BMIs of 35-39.9 and $\geq$40 respectively) (Andreyeva et al., 2004; Arterburn, Maciejewski, & Tsevat, 2005; Elmer, Brown, Nichols, & Oster, 2004; Finkelstein et al., 2008; Finkelstein et al., 2005b; Thompson, Edelsberg, Colditz, Bird, & Oster, 1999; McDonald, Bender, Reffitt, Miller, & Edington, 2006; Quesenberry, Caan, & Jacobson, 1998; Wang et al., 2003; Wee et al, 2005)

Other researchers assessed healthcare costs to the United States economy as a whole. Allison, Zannolli, & Narayan (1999) estimated that obesity may range from as low as 0.89% of annual national healthcare expenditures, up to 4.32%. However, other estimates were higher, including: 5.5% in 1986 (Colditz, 1992), 5.7% in 1995 (Wolf & Colditz, 1998a), 9.1% in 1998 (Finkelstein et al., 2003). One study assessed obesity-related healthcare costs to US businesses at $12.7 billion (Thompson et al., 1998).

Methodology

Researchers used a number of different methods to calculate healthcare costs associated with overweight and obesity. In the case of specific sample populations, researchers measured actual healthcare expenditures from healthcare provider data. In the case of estimates of costs to the economy as a whole, these methods include economic modeling (Allison et al., 1999; Finkelstein et al., 2004) and "Population Attributable Risk" (PAR) Colditz, 1992, 1999; Wolf & Colditz, 1994, 1996, 1998a). Population attributable risk is an epidemiologic method of assessing healthcare costs. Researchers who use this method first determine the costs of certain diseases to the national healthcare spending, then assess the percentage of these costs attributable to obesity and sum these costs. This method may underestimate costs by limiting the number of diseases included in the calculation. Conversely, it may overestimate costs by "double-counting" costs associated with co-morbidities.

Sample Population

Cost estimates of healthcare spending also differed by sample population. In some cases, researchers used nationally representative sample data sourced from nationally collected datasets (Andreyeva et al., 2004; Arterburn et al., 2005; Finkelstein et al., 2008, 2005b; 2004; 2003; Heithoff, Cuffel, Kennedy, & Peters, 1997; Lakdawalla, Goldman, & Shang, 2005; Sturm, 2002; Sturm et al., 2004; Thompson et al., 1999, Thompson et al., 1998; Wee et a;., 2005; Wolf & Colditz, 1998). Other researchers studied convenience samples from health plans, firms, or other organizations (Bungum, Satterwhite, Jackson, & Morrow, 2003; Burton, Chen, Schutz & Edington, 1998; Dall et al., 2007; Elmer et al., 2004; Long & Reed, 2006; Pronk, Goodman, O'Connor, & Martinson, 1999b; Pronk, Tan, & O'Connor, 1999a; Quesenberry et al., 1998; Raebel et al., 2004; Robbins, Robbins, Chao, Russ, & Fonseca ,2002; Thompson et al., 2001, 1999; Wang et al., 2006, 2003). Costs associated with these sample populations were assessed by researchers over time using prospective or retrospective cohort techniques, or by studying cross-sectional associations at a single point in time. Occasionally, researchers estimated healthcare costs associated with obesity using hypothetical cohorts (Gorsky, Pamuk, Williamson, Shaffer, & Koplan, 1996; Oster et al., 2000, Tucker et al., 2006).

Age of Populations Under Study

The majority of studies assessed obesity-related healthcare costs in workers, or persons younger than retirement age. Exceptions include studies that used the population attributable risk method of cost-estimation. Only a few of the studies specifically address older Americans (Lakdawalla et al., 2005; Leigh, Hubert, & Romano, 2005; Sturm et al., 2004).

Temporal Period

Researchers typically assessed the association between weight and healthcare over a relatively short period of time, either a cross-sectional analysis, or in the case of cohort studies, usually no more than 10 years. There were five exceptions to this however: Gorsky et al. (1996) assessed costs for a cohort of middle-aged women over 25 years, and four studies assessed lifetime healthcare costs associated with obesity (Allison et al., 1999; Finkelstein et al., 2008; Thompson et al., 1999; Tucker et al., 2006).

BMI Range Versus Individual BMI Unit

Typically, researchers assessed healthcare costs and weight using accepted BMI ranges, such as ≥30 as a definition of obesity, or 30-34.9 as obesity category I. In a few instances, researchers estimated healthcare cost increases per incremental BMI unit (e.g., the effect of increasing BMI from 31 to 32). Pronk et al., (1999b) found that per BMI unit increased costs 1.9%, for Raebel et al. (2004), the figure was 2.3%, and for Wang et al. (2006) it was 4%. These researchers thus estimated a linear relationship between BMI and healthcare costs, where many other researchers found a J-shaped relationship, as noted above.

Studies Selected for Inclusion in the Model

Two studies were chosen as sources for the model healthcare costing inputs for ages 20-85: Finkelstein et al. (2005), and Andreyeva et al. (2004). No single study provided costing information that was both representative of the US population for all age groups and delineated between the multiple levels of obesity. The age range under study for the Finkelstein article was 18-64. In the model developed here, Finkelstein's figures are used for ages 20-65, and Andreyeva's figures are used for ages 65-85, even though the age range for the Andreyeva study was 54-69. The higher age in the Andreyeva range is not substantially greater than for the Finkelstein study. However, no study was located that assessed healthcare costs for US adults 65-85 and that used nationally representative data, and assessed costs for all three levels of obesity. Medical costs tend to increase with age, and this at least is reflected in the Andreyeva study. It is also likely that the costing inputs for the ages 65-85 in the model derived from the Andreyeva study are conservative, given the age range of the study is 54-69. A study by Lakdawalla et al. (2005) calculated that the lifetime healthcare costs of an obese 70 year old was $39,000 (in 2004 dollars) greater than for a 70 year old of normal weight.

ry Results of Healthcare Costing Studies

	BMI Criteria (kg/m^2)	Study population / Methodology	Summary Results
The ts of	Obesity: BMI ≥ 29	Estimated lifetime healthcare costs of obesity of those aged 20-85 years, using published data and economic modeling	• Healthcare costs attributable to obesity when adjusted f mortality: 0.89-4.32% annual healthcare expenditure

4):
 	
Care
	Normal: 18.5-24.9
	Overweight: 25-29.9
	Obese I: 30-34.9
	Obese II: 35-39.9
	Obese III: ≥ 40
		Data from the 1996, 1998 and 2000 Health and Retirement Study - men and women 54-69 years old. Nationally representative sample. Self-reported height and weight.	**[2002 dollars]**
			• Increased BMI strongly associated with increased healt however the effect was non-linear
			• Increases in healthcare costs compared to normal weigl 25% (obese I), 50% (obese II); 100% (obese III)
			• Healthcare costs/annum of normal weight, overweight, grade II, grade III:
			  • Men: $3915; $4561; $4738; $6179; $8017
			  • Women: $3991; $4365; $5085; $5723; $8440

): esity res	Normal: 18.5-24.9 Overweight: 25-29.9 Obese I: 30-34.9 Obese II: 35-39.9 Obese III: ≥ 40	Data on 16,262 adults in 2000 Medical Expenditure Panel Survey. Nationally representative sample. Cross sectional data analysis	**[2000 dollars]** • Focused on healthcare costs of morbid obesity (obesity • Morbidly obese twice as likely as normal-weight adults healthcare costs in 2000 • Healthcare costs for obesity grade III: 81% ($1975), 65% ($1735), 47% ($1415) and 25% (! than those of normal weight, overweight, obese class class II, respectively • Estimated US healthcare expenditures for morbidly obe Greater than $11billion

'The
Mass
and
	Normal: <25
	Overweight: 25-29.9
	Obese: ≥30
		Survey of 506 city government workers; cross-sectional data analysis	[Note medical claim data available for only 269 study part
			• BMI significantly correlated with healthcares costs, cont gender, race, smoking, and education
			• Overweight and obesity status predict healthcare costs:
			  • Average annual healthcare costs per annum:
			   - Normal weight: $114
			   - Overweight: $573
			   - Obese: $620

	BMI Criteria (kg/m^2)	Study population / Methodology	Summary Results
): "The ody	Obese/"At risk for BMI": ≥ 27.8(men) ≥ 27.3(women)	843 First Chicago NBD employees - medical cost data. Part of a larger study of 3,066 First Chicago NBD employees	• Mean annual healthcare costs for BMI at risk: $6,82 $4,496 • Average annual healthcare costs for BMI ≥30: $10,9 (men) • Average annual healthcare costs over age 45: Women: $10,830 (at risk for BMI); $6,113 (not at Men: $6,192 (at risk for BMI); $3,606 (not at risk
conomic	Obese: BMI ≥ 27.8	Population Attributable Risk	**[1986 dollars]** Diseases included: type 2 diabetes mellitus, cardiovasc bladder disease, hypertension, cancer (breast and colon • Estimated healthcare cost of obesity in US in 1986: $39.3 billion, or 5.5% of US healthcare spending If musculoskeletal disorders included (e.g. osteoa costs would increase to 7.8% of US healthcare sp
conomic nd	Obese: BMI >= 30	Population Attributable Risk	**[1995 dollars]** Diseases included: type 2 diabetes mellitus, hypertensi disease, gall bladder disease, osteoarthritis, cancer (brea endometrium) • Healthcare costs of obesity: - $70 billion, or 7% of
Cost eing ith ohol in the stem's Enrolled	Underweight: <18.5 Normal: 18.5-24.9 Overweight: 25-29.9 Obese I: 30-34.9 Obese II: 35-39.9 Obese III: ≥ 40 Increased active duty normal BMI to 27 due to increased muscularity.	4.3 million participants under 65 in US military health system's TRICARE population in 2006. Cross-sectional data analysis	**[2006 dollars]** • Annual Department of Defense healthcare costs due t obesity: $1.1 billion

	BMI Criteria (kg/m^2)	Study population / Methodology	Summary Results
on	Overweight: 25-29.9 Obese I: 30-34.9 Obese II: 35-39.9 Obese III: ≥ 40	15,174 enrollees in Kaiser Permanente Northwest Division, ages 35-65. Retrospective cohort study over 3 years.	**[1999 dollars]** • Weight gain of ≥ 20lb in 3 year period positively correlat[e] increased healthcare costs • No significant correlation in increased healthcare costs fo[r] gained 5-19lbs, relative to weight-maintainers • Adjusted increased medical care costs for those who gain[e] $561 • Baseline healthcare costs per person: $2317 (overweight) I); $3047 (obese II); $3586 (obese III) • Changes in costs over three years per person: $294 (over[w] (obese I); $460 (obese II); $276 (obese III)

:
)
:
	Overweight: 25-29.9
	Obese: ≥ 30
		1998 Medical Expenditure Panel Survey and 1996-1997 National Health Interview Surveys. Nationally representative data. Cross sectional data analysis	**[2002 dollars]**
			• Overweight and obesity spending in US in 1998: 9.1% of healthcare spending, or $78.5 billion ($92.6 billion in[…]
			• Average annual healthcare spending due to obesity: 37%
			• Estimated average per person increase of being overweig[ht]
			  • Out of pocket, private, Medicaid and Medicare spe[…] $143; $271; $533
			• Estimated average per person increase of being obese: $7[…]
			  • Out of pocket, private, Medicaid and Medicare spe[…] $423; $864; $1486
			• Total medical spending for obesity by insurance (out of p[…] Medicaid and Medicare): 3.9%, 4.7%, 6.7%, 6.5%.
			  • Total: 5.3%

:
of
le
	Obesity: ≥30	1998 Medical Expenditure Panel Survey, 1996-1997 National Health Interview Surveys, and Behavioral Risk Factor Surveillance System (BRFSS) data. Nationally representative data. Cross sectional data analysis	**[2003 dollars]**
			• Medical spending attributable to obesity: $75 billion in 20[…]
			• Percentage of obesity-related medical spending by Medic[…] Medicaid: 50%
			• State estimates, range:
			  • Medicare: $87 million (Wyoming) - $1.7 billion (C[…]
			  • Medicaid: $23 million (Wyoming) - $3.5 billion (C[…]
			Average obesity-related healthcare spending by state: approx[…]

	BMI Criteria (kg/m^2)	Study population / Methodology	Summary Results

(2005): besity e	Normal: 18.5-24.9
	Overweight: 25-29.9
	Obese I: 30-34.9
	Obese II: 35-39.9
	Obese III: ≥ 40
		2000 and 2001 Medical Expenditure Panel Survey data (participants aged 18-64). Econometric analysis. Nationally representative data	[2004 dollars]
			• Estimated costs of healthcare and absenteeism of ol with 1000 employees: $285,000
			• Increased healthcare expenditure over normal weig
			    Women: Overweight - $495; Obese I - $1,071; Obese III - $1,359
			    Men: Overweight - $169; Obese I - $392; Obe: - $1,591

(2008): ledical
 	
Obesity: Obesity
	Normal: 21-24.9
	Overweight: 25-29.9
	Obese I: 30-34.9
	Obese II/III: ≥35
		2001-2004 2000 and 2001 Medical Expenditure Panel Survey data. Lifetime costing estimate, beginning at age 20 and 65	[2007 dollars]
			• Lifetime healthcare costs, adjusting for mortality, positive for white and black men and women
			• Lifetime healthcare costs of overweight are close white women
			• Obese I / Obese II-III healthcare costs
			    Starting age 20:
			    • Men (white, black): $16,490, $12,290 / $16,7
			    • Women (white, black): $21,550, $5,340 / $29
			    Starting age 65:
			    • Men (white, black): $9,940, $19,270 / $20,51
			    • Women (white, black): $17,640, $4,660 / $25

96): "The Care Costs Remain r 40 Years	Non-overweight: 21-24.9 Overweight: 25-28.9 Severely overweight: ≥29	Incidence-based analysis. Three hypothetical cohorts, 10,000 women aged 40-65.	[1990 dollars] • Diseases included: heart disease, hypertension, ty[gallstones and osteoarthritis • Estimated excess costs over 25 years of severely c 10,000 women, compared to non-overweight • Estimated excess costs over 25 years of overweigl women, compared to non-overweight cohort • Estimated excess costs over 25 years of a severely in comparison to one of normal weight: $5,32 • Estimated total in the following 25 years on treatin aged women in US: $16 billion

110

	BMI Criteria (kg/m^2)	Study population / Methodology	Summary Results
"The Body	Overweight ≥27.8 (men) ≥27.3 (women)	1987 National Medical Expenditure Survey data (limited to persons aged 18-65). Cross sectional data analysis	**[1993 dollars]** • Normal weight BMI associated with 6.3% to 36% lowe: healthcare costs (females) and 3.6% to 18.2% lowe • Estimated excess annual costs per overweight person by to person of BMI 22: (BMI of 24, 26, 28, 30, 32, 34, 36, 38, 40): • Women: $131, $271, $418, $575, $742, $919, $1107, $ • Men: $ 51, $104. $158, $213, $249, $265, $279, $293, :
5): sity erly"	Underweight: <20 Normal: 20-24.9 Overweight: 25-29.9 Obese: ≥ 30	Micro-simulation. Data from Medicare Current Beneficiary Survey. Nationally representative sample of Medicare population	**[2004 dollars]** • Obesity is correlated with higher lifetime and annual he • Obese 70 year will incur $39,000 more in costs related that person's lifetime ($36,000 to Medicare, $3,000 • Increased estimated Medicare expenses for 70 year old, year old of normal weight (lifetime): 34-35% • Estimated excess Medicare enrollee's annual healthcare
s sts in	Normal: 22-24 Minimally obese: 30-32	Prospective cohort study - 1323 participants. Analyzed surveys of lifestyle factors (1986-1994) and health utilization (1994-1998) of 68-95 year olds.	**[1994 dollars]** • Annual cost savings of normal weight senior, compared seniors: 32.7%, or $1548
he th	Obese: ≥ 30	Analyzed claims data January 2000-December 2004 of private health plans from 61 employers 24.5 million member months Subjects aged 19-64 years.	**[2004 dollars]** • Non-drug medical expenses due to obesity: 2.8%

	BMI Criteria (kg/m²)	Study population / Methodology	Summary Results
"The ...omic ... in a ...ting"	Non-Obese: <25 Mildly Obese: 25-28.9 Moderately to Severely obese: ≥29	Population Attributable Risk analysis, using modeling and secondary data sources. Estimated healthcare costs for a 1-million person hypothetical healthcare plan aged 35-84 years	**[1996 dollars]** Diseases included: hypertension, hypercholesterolemia, ...mellitus, coronary heart disease, stroke, gallbladder dis... of the knee, endometrial cancer • Estimated annual healthcare costs for hypothetical 1... healthcare plan, ages 35-84, due to obesity: $34... of healthcare spending on the diseases included

...(1998): ...ervices ...are Costs ...of a ...e	Reference: 20-24.9
	Obese I: 30-34.9
	Obese II&III: ≥35
		17,118 participants in health survey of a large HMO and direct healthcare costs of these members in 1993	• Healthcare assessed: outpatient visits and costs, inpa... radiology, laboratory and pharmaceutical costs
			• Strong correlation between BMI and healthcare cost... slightly J-shaped
			• Rates of healthcare costs relative to BMI (reference relative rate, obese II/III relative rate):
			  - Ages 20-39: $ 970, 1.24, 1.48
			  - Ages 40-59: $1752, 1.59, 1.72
			  - Ages 60-74: $3086, 1.18, 1.38
			  - Ages ≥75: $4460, 1.04, 0.53
			  - All Ages: $2090, 1.25, 1.44
			
			• The association with obesity and diabetes, hypertens... heart disease largely accounted for the associati... and healthcare costs, but not completely

...Connor, ...Fitness, ...Health	Low risk: <27.8 (men) <27.3 (women) High-risk: ≥27.8 (men) ≥27.3 (women)	8822 members of Midwestern health plan - 1993-1996. Analysis of healthcare and survey data.	• Linear correlation between BMI and medical costs • Medical costs (adjusted for age, chronic conditions) 25, 27-29, 30-34, 35-39, ≥) • $1761, $1638, $1890, $1975, $2091, $2282.
...: ...veen ...Risks ...alth-		5689 members of a Minnesota health plan. Analysis of healthcare and survey data.	• Median health expenditure $600 per person • A 1 unit increase in BMI increased median health ca...

	BMI Criteria (kg/m^2)	Study population / Methodology	Summary Results

and	Normal 18.5-24.9; <u>Overweight and Obese</u> 27.9-68.6	Members of Kaiser Permanente of Colorado healthcare plan. Records on healthcare data on 539 obese and 1225 non-obese individuals, matched for age, sex, SES and chronic disease. Analyzed data from Jan 1- Dec 31, 1998.	• Obese persons had increased: prescription medications drug costs, hospitalization and healthcare costs ove person of normal weight
			• Total annual medical costs
			  • <u>Obese:</u> $585.44
			  • <u>Non-obese:</u> $333.24
			• Medical cost difference between obese and non-obese cost of prescriptions
			• Each unit increase in BMI correlated with 2.3% increas costs
			• Individual with BMI of 40 spends $115 more on medic person with BMI 25, controlling for age, sex + chr
			• Each chronic disease for an obese person costs on avera extra.

y ir	US Military standard 'Maximum Allowable Weight (MAW): <u>MAW BMI men:</u> 27.9 <u>MAW BMI women:</u> 25	4,974 persons aged 17-60 enrolled in active duty managed health care plan. Retrospective cohort analysis.	• In 1997, 20.4% men and 20.5% women in the US Air Fc over allowable limit. • Healthcare costs associated with this excess weight: $19 of annual Air Force medical costs)

	BMI Criteria (kg/m^2)	Study population / Methodology	Summary Results

):
y Rates
nds"
	Underweight: <18.5
	Normal: 18.5-24.9
	Overweight: 25-29.9
	Moderately obese: 30-34.9
	Severely obese: ≥35
		Analyzed data from Health and Retirement Study and Behavioral Risk Factor Surveillance Survey, 1985-2000, 50-69 year olds. Cross-sectional data analysis	**[1992 dollars]**
			• Increased healthcare costs above normal weight (ov… severely obese) 1985-2000
			  • Men: 12.7%; 17.5%, 67%.
			  • Women: 10.5%, 31% and 59.6%
			• Average increase in medical costs of men and wome… severe obesity over those of normal weight - 19…
			• <u>Men:</u> Estimated average costs of healthcare related t… 1990, 1995, 2000, 2005, 2010, 2015, 2020)
			  • $5,656, $5,692, $5,762, $5,837, $5,918, $6,00…
			• <u>Women:</u> Estimated average costs of healthcare relat… 1990, 1995, 2000, 2005, 2010, 2015, 2020)
			  • $5,635, $5,701, $5,772, $5,850, $5,933, $6,02…
			• <u>Men:</u> Estimated excess costs of healthcare related to… normal weight (1985, 1990, 1995, 2000, 2005, …
			  • 10.2%, 11.5%, 12.8%, 14.3%, 15.9%, 17.6%,…
			• <u>Women:</u> Estimated excess costs of healthcare relate… normal weight (1985, 1990, 1995, 2000, 2005, …
			  • 8.6%, 9.8%, 11.2%, 12.7%, 14.3%, 16.1%, 17…

e Effects ng, And cal ts,"	Underweight: <18.5 Normal: 18.5-24.9 Overweight: 25-29.9 Obese: ≥30	1997-1998 Healthcare for Communities - national household phone survey. Subjects aged 18-65. Cross-sectional data analysis.	• BMI is a 'highly significant predictor' of poor physic… disease • BMI has a similar association with poor health as th… years, but a much greater correlation with poor … effects of poverty, smoking or heavy drinking • Obesity is correlated with a 36% greater spending o… outpatient services, and 77% higher spending o… • Increased costs of inpatient and ambulatory care: $3… related to obesity (smoking: $230, problem alcc… $150)

114

	BMI Criteria (kg/m^2)	Study population / Methodology	Summary Results
: A	Normal: 20-24.9 Overweight: 25-29.9 Obese: ≥30	Retrospective cohort study. 1286 members of Kaiser Permanente Northwest Division, HMO in Portland Oregon. Aged 35-64, BMI ≥20, for 9 years, 1990-1998.	**[1998 dollars]** • Normal BMI: Average annual cost of prescription drugs, services, inpatient care, all medical care: • $261, $848, $532 and $1631 respectively. • Cost ratios of above costs for overweight compared to nor 1.37, 0.96, 1.2 and 1.38 • Cost ratios of above costs for obese compared to normal 1.14, 1.10, 1.36 • Total average healthcare costs over the nine year period: (normal), $18,484 (overweight), $21,711 (obese)

s	Non-obese: 22.5
	Mildly Obese: 27.5
	Moderately Obese: 32.5
	Severely Obese: 37.5
		National Health And Nutrition Survey (NHANES) III, Framingham Heart Study and other secondary sources. Longitudinal, lifetime costing model based on disease risk	**[1996 dollars]**
			Diseases included: hypertension, hypercholesterolemia, type mellitus, coronary heart disease, stroke
			• Disease risk significantly higher with increasing BMI.
			• Total discounted lifetime medical costs higher by $10,00(
			• Increases in BMI lowered life expectancy.
			• Costs for men (non-, mildly, moderately and severely obe
			  • 35-44 years: $16,200, $20,200, $25,300, $31,700
			  • 45-54 years: $19,600, $24,000, $29,600, $36,500
			  • 55-64 years: $22,000, $31,200, $37,400
			• Costs for women (non-, mildly, moderately and severely
			  • 35-44 years: $15,200, $18,900, $23,800, $29,700
			  • 45-54 years: $18,800, $23,200, $28,700, $35,300
			  • 55-64 years: $21,900, $26,500, $32,200, $39,000

:	Normal: <25 Mildly Obese: 25-28.9 Moderately or Severely Obese: ≥ 29	Population Attributable Risk. Data sources: NHIS, BLS and other agencies, published literature. Focused on employees aged 25-64	Diseases included: Coronary heart disease, hypertension, typ mellitus, hypercholesterolemia, stroke, gall bladder disease, osteoarthritis, endometrial cancer • Obesity (includes mildly and moderately/severely obese le responsible for 43% of medical care expenditure by U on diseases listed. • Cost to US businesses: $12.7 billion - $2.6 billion mild obe billion for moderately or severe obesity • Aggregate health insurance expenditures on selected diseas obesity: $7.7 billion

	BMI Criteria (kg/m^2)	Study population / Methodology	Summary Results
6): Healthcare Jnit Body ;ase"	Underweight: <17 Normal: 18-24.9 Overweight: 25-29.9 Obese I: 30-34.9 Obese II: 35-39.9 Obese III: ≥ 40	35,932 participants in an indemnity/PPO plan 2001-2002. Examined health survey and claims data. Cross sectional data analysis	**[2004 dollars]** • J-shaped relationship between BMI and healthcar₍ • Between BMI of 25-45, per BMI unit, medical co: (4%) and pharmaceutical costs increased $82 age and gender) • Average amount paid in normal BMI group: $275 $1179 for drug claims • Increase of 4% medical and 7% drug costs /BMI ι
3): "The ween Lung, and veight Concurrent ι a "opulation"	Underweight: <18.5 Normal: 18.5-24.9 Overweight: 25-29.9 Obese I: 30-34.9 Obese II: 35-39.9 Obese III: ≥ 40	177,971 employees and dependents of General Motors Corporation, aged 19 or older, in an indemnity/PPO plan 1996-1997. Health survey and claims data. Height/weight 89% self-reported. Cross-sectional data analysis	**[2000 dollars]** • J-shaped relationship between BMI and healthcar₍ • Median healthcare costs correlated with the BMI ᵨ categories: • Underweight: $3184 • Normal: $2225 • Overweight: $2388 • Obese I: $2801 • Obese II: $3182 • Obese III: $3753
) "Health ιes Obesity lts: ge and	Underweight: <18.5 Normal: 18.5-24.9 Overweight: 25-29.9 Obese I: 30-34.9 Obese II: 35-39.9 Obese III: ≥40	1998 Medical Expenditure Panel Survey. Study population: 11,212 subjects over age 18. Cross sectional data analysis	**[2003 dollars]** • Average annual healthcare spending: $2,970 (norι (overweight), $4,333 (obese) • Average annual healthcare spending (white wome $2128 (normal weight), $2358 (overweight), ΄ $3058 (obese II), $3506 (obese III) • Median unadjusted healthcare spending: $883 (un (normal weight), $744 (overweight), $1092 (₍ II), $1422 (obese III) • Variation in BMI and healthcare costs is associate large increases seen in white and older adults, aged under 35

	BMI Criteria (kg/m²)	Study population / Methodology	Summary Results
8): the esity	Lean: <20 for gallbladder disease,<21 for coronary heart disease, <22 for type 2 diabetes mellitus and colon cancer, <23 for hypertension Obese: ≥29	Population Attributable Risk, and 1988 and 1994 National Health Interview Survey data of persons aged 17-64. Nationally representative. Cross sectional data analysis.	[1995 dollars] Diseases included: Type 2 diabetes mellitus, coronary hea hypertension, gallbladder disease, cancer (breast, endometr osteoarthritis • Total (direct and indirect) costs of obesity in 1995: $99.2 • Total direct medical costs 1995 in US: $51.64 billion, or National Health Expenditure • 63% of direct costs of obesity due to costs associated wit mellitus
6): ht in	Reference: <22 High Normal: 23-24.9 Overweight: 25-29.9 Obese: ≥30	Population Attributable Risk	[1993 dollars] • Diseases included: type 2 diabetes mellitus, coronary hea hypertension, gallbladder disease • Excess healthcare costs associated with obesity in the Un $22.62 billion
4): The	Obesity: ≥27.8 men ≥27.3 women	Population Attributable Risk	[1990 dollars] Diseases included: Type 2 diabetes mellitus, gallbladder d cardiovascular disease, cancer, musculoskeletal disease • Healthcare costs associated with obesity in US in 1990:

Absenteeism Costing

Moving from healthcare costing to studies that estimated obesity-related costs of

absenteeism, Table 4.2 displays a summary of the 17 located studies that assessed

obesity-related absenteeism costs. The studies generally show that absenteeism is

positively correlated with BMI. Cawley, Rizzo and Haas (2007) estimated, for example,

that absenteeism related to obesity may account for 9% of all absenteeism in the United

States, and cost the US economy $4.3 billion per annum. The studies that assessed costs

at the individual level and used greater granularity in the BMI categories in their analysis

—Dall et al., 2007 and Finkelstein et al., 2005b— showed a J-shaped relationship

between weight and absenteeism. One exception to the positive correlation between BMI

and absenteeism and weight was the study by Gates, Succop, Brehm, Gillespie, and

Sommers (2008), which had a small sample size and included normal and underweight in

the same category. The studies in Table 4.2 differed in their units of analysis,

methodology, sample representativeness and temporal period of the study, which are

described in turn below. This is followed by a discussion of the article used to provide

absenteeism-related costs to the Markov model developed for this dissertation.

Unit of Analysis

Researchers most often assessed absenteeism costs and obesity at the individual-level,

rather than the population-level (Bertera, 1991; Bungum et al., 2003; Burtin et al., 1998,

1999; Dall et al, 2007; Finkelstein et al., 2005b; Gates et al., 2008; Ricci & Chee, 2005).

However, researchers also assessed costs at the population level (Cawley et al., 2007;

Klarenbach, Padwal, Chuck, & Jacobs, 2006; Narbro et al., 1999; Robbins et al., 2002;

Thompson et al., 1998; Tsai, Ahmed, Wendt, Bhojani, & Donnelly, 2008; Tucker, Palmer, Valentine, Roze, & Ray, 1998; Wolf, 1998).

Methodology

Absenteeism related to obesity was generally assessed using cross-sectional data analysis of surveys and healthcare data. Exceptions to this included using the population attributable risk method (Thompson et al., 1998; Wolf and Colditz 1998), retrospective cohort analysis (Robbins, 2002) and economic modeling (Cawley 2007; Finkelstein 2005).

Sample Representation

Most researchers assessed absenteeism and health information for sample populations that were not representative of the United States population. Exceptions to this included Cawley et al., 2007; Finkelstein et al., 2005b; Thomspon et al., 1998; and Wolf and Colditz, 1998.

Temporal Period

Most researchers assessed the association between obesity and absenteeism at a single point in time, with a few exceptions. Narbro et al., (1996) Robbins et al. (2002) and Tsai et al. (2008) assessed absenteeism for their sample longitudinally.

Study Selected for Inclusion in the Markov Model

The study results selected for inclusion in the lifetime costing model was Finkelstein et al., (2005). This was the only study located in the obesity costing meta-analysis, shown in Table 4.2 that measured the cost of absenteeism using three levels of obesity, and used nationally representative data in its analysis. The Finkelstein study reported lower than expected costs for the severely obese for both men and women. This may reflect sampling issues of the severely obese working population in the study itself. However, it suggests also that the costing estimates used in the model developed for this dissertation may be conservative.

Country	BMI Criteria (kg/m²)	Study sample/ methodology	Summary Results
United States	Overweight/obesity: "20% more than ideal"	46,000 employees from DuPont United States workforce. Cross-sectional data analysis of survey and observational data	• Excess illness days for overweight: 0.36 • Annual illness costs excess: $400.60 per person

United States	Normal: < 25
	Overweight: 25-29.9
	Obese: ≥ 30
		Survey of 506 city government workers; cross-sectional data analysis	[Note absenteeism information available on 487 of st participants]
			• BMI significantly correlated with absence, controll gender, race, smoking, education.
			• Overweight and obesity status predict absence cost
			  • Average absent hours per year:
			    BMI <25: 27.21
			    BMI 25-29.9: 30.35
			    BMI 30+: 35.52

United States	Not available	564 employees (telephone customer service representatives) of First Card, a credit card issuer. Analyzed company health records, productivity data	• Illness absence (including short term disability) in associated with BMI
			• Average illness absence hours lost per week:
			  Total population: 0.6
			  BMI at risk: 0.8

United States	'At risk for BMI':
	≥ 27.8 (men)
	≥ 27.3 (women)
		3,066 employees of First Chicago NBD employees; cross sectional analysis of employee health data	• Average sick days per year:
			  At risk for BMI 8.45 sick days/year
			  Not at risk for BMI 3.73 sick days/year
			• Costs/annum (cost per sick day: $189):
			  At risk for BMI: $1,546 per person
			  Not at risk $683 per person
			  Average cost per person for at risk for BMI: $8

	Country	BMI Criteria (kg/m^2)	Study sample/ methodology	Summary Results
07): cific sts bid	United States	Underweight: < 18.5 Healthy: 18-5-24.9 Overweight: 25-29.9 Obese: 30-39.9 Morbidly obese: ≥ 40	Medical Expenditure Panel Survey data 2000-2004. Cross sectional data analysis. Nationally representative data.	[2004 dollars] • Annual absenteeism costs correlated with ob $4.3 billion • Up to 9% of the total nationwide cost of abs obesity • Absenteeism related to obesity varies by occ • Overall likelihood of missing work greater t weight: Overweight 32%; obese 61%; • Incremental per employee costs from absen obesity and morbid obesity: Women: obese - $142; morbidly obese Men: obesity - $70; morbidly obese - $
"Cost Being With lcohol nd thin th RE	United States	Underweight: <18.5 Normal: 18.5-24.9 Overweight: 25-29.9 Obese I: 30-34.9 Obese II: 35-39.9 Obese III: ≥ 40 (Increased active duty normal BMI to 27 due to increased muscularity)	4.3 million participants under 65 in military health system TRICARE population in 2006. Cross-sectional data analysis	[2006 dollars] • Absenteeism costs (overweight or obese): 6 Employee (FTE) days lost; Equivalent million • Days absent (active duty personnel aged 21 Normal weight: 4.2 Overweight: 6 Obesity I: 8 Obesity II and III combined:12.2
sts of Full-	United States	Normal: 18.5-24.9 Overweight: 25-29.9 Obese I: 30-34.9 Obese II: 35-39.9 Obese III: ≥ 40	2001 and 2002 National Health Interview Survey data (participants aged 18-64). Econometric analysis. Nationally representative data.	[2004 dollars] • Missed number of work days per year: Women: Normal - 3.4; Overweight -3. II - 6.4; Obese III - 8.2 Men: Normal - 3; Overweight -3; Obes Obese III - 5 • Increased costs over normal weight: Women: Overweight - $93; Obese I - $ Obese III - $805 Men: Overweight - $6; Obese I - $70; (III - $436

Country	BMI Criteria (kg/m^2)	Study sample/ methodology	Summary Results
United States	Normal: <25 Overweight: 25-29.9 Mildly Obese: 30-34.9 Moderately or Extremely Obese: ≥ 35	341 employees from 8 mid-size manufacturing companies in Kentucky. Survey and other employee data. Cross sectional data analysis.	• Arithmetic mean of absenteeism (hours): Normal 63.76 Overweight - 26.86; Mildly Obese: 91.08 Moderately or Extremely Obese: - 73.48 • Annual absenteeism cost for moderately or extre workers (using $21.44 average hourly wage) greater than absenteeism costs for all other e study combined)
Canada	Normal: 18.5-24.9 Overweight: 25-29.9 Obese I: 30-34.9 Obese II: 35-39.9 Obese III: ≥ 40	Representative sub-sample aged 20-59 from 2000 to 2001 Canadian Community Health Survey. Cross-sectional data analysis	**[2004 Canadian dollars]** • Examined "workforce participation" - defined by absenteeism + employment. • Workforce participation was lower for difference obesity, even when adjusting for other factor demographics, education and other chronic h • Participation in workforce was inversely related t • Odds Ratio of workforce participation (reference Obesity I: 0.97; Obesity II: 0.86; Obesity III • Odds Ratio of absenteeism (reference – normal w 1.15; Obesity II: 1.15; Obesity III: 1.24 • Cost of workforce non-participation due to obesit estimated to be C$187 million in 2004
Sweden	Obese: ≥28	Retrospective study of 1298 obese persons aged 30-59 years.	**[1994 Swedish Krona (SEK)]** • Annual number of sick leave days positively corr obesity • Over one year, the obese cohort under study had higher sick leave than the general Swedish p • Cost of sick-leave for obese cohort (1106 persons non-obese population: 13.1 million SEK • Total estimated extra cost of sick leave for the ob 1988: 1.1billion SEK

	Country	BMI Criteria (kg/m²)	Study sample/ methodology	Summary Results
en and y"	United States	Normal: <27 Overweight: 27-29.9 Obese: 30-39.9 Extremely Obese: ≥ 40	683 employees of three managed care health plans and American Airlines. Survey data.	• Severe obesity was correlated with a higher r work lost in the previous 30 days
005): ime xcess	United States	Underweight: <18 Normal: 18-24.9 Overweight: 25-29.9 Obese: ≥ 30	6894 respondents to the Caremark American Productivity Audit, a national telephone survey on work productivity and health. Survey respondents were workers aged 18-65. Nationally representative. Cross sectional data analysis.	[2002 dollars] • Estimated excess cost of absenteeism of obese that of workers of normal weight: $3.8 bi • Cost of absenteeism per obese worker: $537 [Cost per obese worker of absenteeism + produc of the cost, therefore estimated cost of absentee $537]
2): ody tive S	United States	US Military standard 'Maximum Allowable Weight (MAW): MAW BMI men: 27.9; MAW BMI women: 25	4,974 persons aged 17-60 enrolled in active duty managed health care plan. Retrospective cohort analysis.	• In 1997, 20.4% men and 20.5% women in the weights over allowable limit. • Estimated lost workdays due to excess weight • Estimated cost of lost workdays due to excess
	United States	Normal: <25 Mildly Obese: 25-28.9 Moderately or Severely Obese: ≥ 29	Population Attributable Risk. Data sources: National Health Interview Survey data; Bureau of Labor Statistics data and from other agencies; published literature. Focused on employees aged 25-64	Diseases included: CHD, hypertension, type 2 d hypercholesterolemia, stroke, gall bladder disea osteoarthritis, endometrial cancer. • Aggregate obesity-attributable expenditure on US businesses: • Paid sick leave: $2.4 billion

	Country	BMI Criteria (kg/m^2)	Study sample/ methodology	Summary Results

e
 	
of
	United States	Normal: 18.5-24.9
		Overweight: 25-29.9
		Obese: ≥30
			4153 employees from Shell oil. Analyzed internal healthcare system data, 1994-2003. Prospective study, objectively measured data. Excluded absences less than 6 days.	• Compared with normal weight employees, obese
				  • 80% more likely to be absent (24.0 compare workers)
				  • Absent 3.7 more days per year (7.7 compare
				• Increase in obesity prevalence in study sample 1! 42%
				• Estimated direct cost of illness absence per year company: $11,166,250,
				• : $1,873,500 (overweight and obese employees)
				• Estimated illness absence due to obesity:
				  • 1994: 31%
				  • 2003: 36%

of	United States	Percent body-fat from skinfold tests. Lean: ≤15% men, ≤20% women. Average: 15.1%-24.9% men, 20.1-29.9% women Obese: ≥25% for men; ≥30% or more for women. Cross sectional data analysis.	10,825 employees of 50 different companies at Health Advancement Services Inc. Cross sectional data analysis	• Obesity significantly correlated with high and m absenteeism • Obese were 1.74 and 1.61 times more likely to e days in last 6 months) and moderate (3-6 da months) levels of absenteeism respectively • Excess costs of high and moderate absenteeism obese versus lean workers: $128,600 per 10(

	Country	BMI Criteria (kg/m²)	Study sample/ methodology	Summary Results
ed	United States	Obese: ≥27.3 (women) ≥27.8 (men)	Population Attributable Risk. 1988 and 1994 National Health Interview Survey data of personal aged 17-64. Nationally representative. Cross sectional data analysis.	**[1995 dollars]** Diseases included: Type 2 diabetes mellitus, cc hypertension, gallbladder disease, cancer (breas colon), osteoarthritis • Cost of lost productivity (lost work days) in 1 $3.9Billion, 39.2 million days of work. • Increase between 1988 and 1994 of work-lost • 70% of lost work days due to obese women • Work days lost due to obesity in 1988: 52,59 • Cost of work days lost due to obesity in 1988 • Work days lost due to obesity in 1994: 58,45(• Cost of work days lost due to obesity in 1994

Disability Insurance/Retirement

Having discussed obesity-related healthcare and absenteeism costing studies, this section

reports on the obesity-related disability insurance/retirement. Nine studies were located

that assessed the likelihood of disability insurance due to obesity. All of these studies

were from Nordic countries, which may reflect easier access to national-level datasets.

The term "disability retirement" and "disability pension" are used by many of these

studies. These terms are used interchangeably with "disability insurance". All of the

studies in this section show that disability retirement and obesity are positively

correlated. Studies with greater granularity of obesity cutoff rates tend to show a J-shaped

relationship between disability retirement and obesity. The studies differed in their units

of analysis, methodology, sample representativeness and temporal period of the study,

which are described in turn below. This is followed by a discussion of the article used to

provide disability-related costs to the Markov model developed for this dissertation.

Most studies assessed disability insurance associated with obesity in terms of the odds

ratio or relative risk, at the individual level. Researchers typically assessed disability

retirement costs associated with obesity using cohort analyses. None of the studies

reviewed in this section assessed a population that was representative of the US

population. Rather, most sample populations were nationally representative of the

Nordic countries of Finland, Sweden and Denmark. In contrast to many of the other

obesity costing studies presented in this chapter, and in keeping with cohort study design,

most of the studies analyzing disability retirement assessed the association over an

extended period. This is likely due to the nature of the phenomenon under study; it takes time for the effect under study (in this case disability) to manifest and impact the individual to the point that they join disability insurance rolls.

Study Selected for Inclusion in the Markov Model

No specific study was selected for inclusion in the Markov model from the articles summarized here. Rather, the studies informed the probability of receiving disability insurance. According to the costing studies that summarized in Table 4.4, estimates of the impact of obesity on the likelihood of receiving a disability pension in Scandinavian countries ranges from 35% increased risk for those with BMI $\geq$30 (Karnehed et al., 2007) to over 300% for those of BMI $\geq$35 (Neovius et al., 2008). As there has been little work on this estimated impact in the US, and it is likely that Scandinavian benefits are more generous than in the US (perhaps providing greater incentive to join disability insurance rolls), these probabilities were estimated conservatively at a 10% increased risk for people whose BMI is 30-34.9 and 30% increased risk for people whose BMIs are $\geq$35. The association between obesity and disability insurance in the US may be a fruitful area for future research.

ry of Disability Retirement /Disability Insurance Studies

	Country	BMI Criteria (kg/m^2)	Study population / Methodology	Summary Results
y	Denmark	Reference: ≤20 Obese: >27	892 persons from general population, retrospective cohort analysis between years 1977 and 1992	• In Demark, 0.625% of the population begin disability pe every year (20,000 people from population of 3.2 milli • Odds Ratio of receiving disability pension with BMI >2
t,	Denmark	Normal: <25 Overweight: 25-29.9 Obese: ≥30	12,028 nurses over the age of 44. Survey and longitudinal disability data from national registry. Objectively measured height and weight.	• 11% had entered disability pension by age 66 • Overweight increased the risk of disability pension, haza disability pension if obese: 1.12 • Obesity increased the risk of disability pension, hazard r pension if obese: 1.63
:	Sweden	Underweight: <18.5 Normal: 18.5-24.9 Overweight: 25-29.9 Obese: ≥30	366,929 Swedish men born 1952-59. Swedish Military Service Conscription Register, Longitudinal Database of Education, Income and Occupation, Hospital Discharge Register and Cause of Death Register. Retrospective cohort analysis.	• 3.8% men received disability pension during the follow- • Compared to those who were normal weight at age 18, w country of birth, city, parental education, marital status and other factors, the hazard ratios for those who were obese were 1.03 and 1.35 respectively. Thus, at age 1 risk of later disability pension was 35% higher than fo normal weight. • J-Shaped relationship between risk of disability pension

	Country	BMI Criteria (kg/m^2)	Study population / Methodology	Summary Results
o en tus, and ed	Sweden	Obese: ≥30	5313 subjects (males aged 48) prospective cohort study. Follow-up period: 11 years.	• Initiated disability pension during follow-up period: 1[...] • Relative risk of disability pension for obesity: 2.0

96): and in - ns"	Sweden	Underweight: <20
		 Normal: 20-24.99
		 Overweight: 25-29.99
		 Obese: ≥30
			5313 subjects (males aged 48) prospective cohort study. Follow-up period: 11 years. Objectively measured height and weight.	• Adjusting for smoking status, there was a J-shaped re[...] BMI and disability pension
				 • Relative risk of disability pension:
				   - Overweight: 1.3
				   - Obese: 2.8
				 • Rates of disability pension during follow-up period:
				   - Underweight: 18.8%
				   - Normal: 9.9%
				   - Overweight: 12.6%
				   - Obese: 23.9%

): ick- se	Sweden	Obese: ≥28	Retrospective study of 1298 obese persons aged 30-59 years. Data from Swedish National Social Insurance Board	**[1994 Swedish Krona (SEK)]** • Disability pension was 2.0-2.8 times greater in the obes[...] general population • Disability pension was 2.3 to 3.9 times greater for obes[...] ≥40 than the general Swedish female population • Cost of disability pension for obese cohort (1298 perso[...] non-obese population: 15.0 million SEK • Estimated annual disability pension costs for 100 obese[...] for non-obese persons: 0.4-2.5 million SEK • Total estimated extra cost of disability pension for the [...] 1988: 2.5 billion SEK

Country	BMI Criteria (kg/m^2)	Study population / Methodology	Summary Results
Sweden	Underweight: <18.5 Normal: 18.5-24.9 Overweight: 25-29.9 Moderately Obese: 30-34.9 Morbidly Obese: ≥35	Swedish Military Service Conscription Registry 1969-1994; Cause of Death Registry; Multi-Generation registry' Population of Housing Censuses and the Registry of the Total Population; Social Insurance Office. Retrospective cohort analysis.	• 60,024 subjects granted disability pension in 28.4 millio follow-up • Risks of disability pension correlated significantly with obesity in young adulthood - J-shaped relationship bet risk of disability pension • Hazard ratios of future disability pension in young adult those of normal weight (=1): - Overweight: 1.36 - Moderately Obese: 1.87 - Morbidly Obese: 3.04 • Hazard ratios of future disability pension in young adult psychiatric causes (e.g. circulatory, musculoskeletal, t compared to those of normal weight (=1): - Overweight: 1.48 - Moderately Obese: 2.19 Morbidly Obese: 3.68
Finland	<22.5 22.5-24.9 25-27.4 27.5-29.9 30-32.4 ≥ 32.5 Obese: ≥30	12,053 female and 19,076 male workers, aged 25-64 at baseline. Social Insurance Institution of Finland data 1966-1972, through 1982. Prospective cohort study	• New cases of disability pension in cohort during follow- • BMI linearly and highly correlated with early work disa • Controlling for age, region, occupation and tobacco use, work disability of BMI : ≥30 over BMI <22.5: - Men: 1.5 - Women: 2.0 • Overall early disability pension caused by BMI ≥30: - Men: 4% - Women: 10% • Higher risk of disability pension due to higher incidence morbidity
Finland	Underweight: <18.5 Normal: <18.8-24.9 Overweight: 25-29.9 Obese: ≥ 30	Representative cohort of 19,518 Finnish adults aged 20-92 years. Follow-up period: 15 years.	• Obese men (non-smokers) aged 20-64 experienced 0.63 m disability pension than men of normal weight. Obese r women experienced 0.52 more years.

Productivity Costing

A total of four studies were located that assess the productivity costs associated with obesity. These studies are summarized in Table 4.4. Please note that several of the studies use the term "presenteeism" to indicate loss of productivity due to weight/health. Ricci (2005), offers perhaps the most detailed explanation of the productivity loss associated with weight, describing it as: "the average amount of time between arriving at work and starting work on days when a worker is not feeling well and the average frequency of engaging in five specific work behaviors (i.e., losing concentration, repeating a job, working more slowly than usual, feeling fatigued at work, and doing nothing at work)" (p. 1228). Collectively, the productivity studies show an inverse correlation between BMI and productivity. The studies differed in their units of analysis, methodology, sample representativeness and temporal period of the study, which are described in turn below. This is followed by a discussion of the article used to provide absenteeism-related costs to the Markov model developed in the present study.

Three of the studies (Burton et al., 1999; Gates et al., 2008; Ricci & Chee, 2005) assessed productivity costs associated with obesity on an individual basis. Dall et al. (2007), on the other hand, estimated productivity costs associated with obesity in the population as a whole. Only one of the studies (Burton et al,, 1999) objectively measured productivity, by studying call throughput in telephone customer service representatives. The other studies relied on self-reported productivity measures, such as survey responses regarding perceived productivity. Only one study (Ricci and Chee, 2005) assessed nationally representative data. The other studies assessed data on convenience population samples.

Study Selected for Inclusion in the Markov Model

Only one study (Ricci and Chee, 2005) analyzed costing information related to

productivity used nationally representative data. Therefore, the costs determined by Ricci

were used as inputs to the Markov model.

nmary of Productivity Costing Studies

	Country	BMI Criteria (kg/m²)	Study population / Methodology	Summary Results
)9): lth er	United States	Not available	564 employees (telephone customer service representatives) of First Card, a credit card issuer. Analyzed company health records, productivity data. Productivity objectively measured	• Productivity (absenteeism, disability and ' inversely associated with BMI • Average productivity hours lost per week: <u>Total population</u>: 3.82 <u>BMI at risk</u>: 4.98
Being With cohol nd thin th RE	United States	<u>Underweight</u>: <18.5 <u>Normal</u>: 18.5-24.9 <u>Overweight</u>: 25-29.9 <u>Obese I</u>: 30-34.9 <u>Obese II</u>: 35-39.9 <u>Obese III</u>: ≥ 40 (Increased active duty normal BMI to 27 due to increased muscularity)	4.3 million participants under 65 in military health system TRICARE population in 2006. Cross-sectional data analysis. Productivity ('presenteeism') based on self-reported data.	**[2006 dollars]** • Presenteeism (reduced performance): Full days: 17,000 - $2.6 million annually
3): le Mass ace	United States	<u>Normal</u>: <25 <u>Overweight</u>: 25-29.9 <u>Mildly Obese</u>: 30-34.9 <u>Moderately or Extremely Obese</u>: ≥ 35	341 employees from 8 mid-size manufacturing companies in Kentucky. Survey and other employee data. Cross sectional data analysis.	• <u>Productivity loss (%)</u>: Normal/underweight: 3.25 Overweight: 3.13 Mildly Obese: 2.45 Moderately or Extremely Obese: 4.16 • Annual productivity cost for moderately or workers (using $21.44 average hourly greater than absenteeism costs for all o study combined)

Country	BMI Criteria (kg/m^2)	Study population / Methodology	Summary Results

United States	Underweight: <18
	Normal: 18-24.9
	Overweight: 25-29.9
	Obese: ≥ 30
		6894 respondents to the Caremark American Productivity Audit, a national telephone survey on work productivity and health. Survey respondents were workers aged 18-65. Nationally representative. Cross sectional data analysis	**[2002 dollars]**
			• Productivity was inversely correlated with obesit
			• Percentage of US workforce reporting absenteeis productivity related to health:
			  - Normal: 36.4%
			  - Overweight: 34.7%
			  - Obese: 42.3%
			• Average absenteeism and lost productivity time r per week:
			  - Normal: 4.2
			  - Overweight: 4.2
			  - Obese: 4.8
			• Estimated excess cost of productivity of obese U that of workers of normal weight: $7.84 billi
			• Cost per obese worker: $1627 (absenteeism plus presenteeism/productivity). [Presenteeism: 6 therefore cost per obese worker: $1,090]

Other Costing Studies

Several other studies were located in the literature search that suggested other external costs associated with obesity. These other costs include workers' compensation (Østbye, Dement, & Krause, 2007), private disability insurance and life insurance (Thompson et al., 1998), fuel consumption (Jacobsen and McLay, 2006) and child safety (Trifiletti et al., 2006), which are discussed in turn below. Summaries of a subset of these studies are provided in Table 4.5.

Workers Compensation: Using a retrospective cohort study design, Østbye et al. (2007) found a positive, J-shaped correlation between indemnity claims costs and weight in members of a university healthcare organization.

Private Disability Insurance and Life Insurance: Thompson (1998) calculated disability insurance and life insurance costs to US businesses using a population attributable risk method. Results from the study showed that obesity-related costs to US businesses for life insurance and disability insurance were $1.8 billion and $800 million, respectively.

Fuel Consumption: The increase in obesity rates may also affect fuel consumption. Jacobsen and McLay (2006) estimated that compared to obesity rates in 1960, annual fuel consumption for cars and trucks in the United States was 938 million gallons greater in 2002. Dannenberg, Burton and Jackson (2004) provided estimates of the impact of obesity on airlines, calculating that for the year 2000, the rise in obesity rates increased consumption of jet fuel by 350 million gallons, which cost approximately $275 million.

However, this commentary by Dannenberg et al. was not included in Table 4.5 as it was not a peer-reviewed article.

Child Safety: A study by Trifiletti et al. (2006) found that child safety may be another indirect cost of the rise in obesity rates in children. In an analysis of automobile child safety seats and weight status of children, Trifiletti et al. found that approximately 285,000 children in the United States in 2005 would have difficulty in finding appropriate safety seats due to their weight.

Studies Selected for Inclusion in the Model

None of the costs summarized in Table 4.5 were included in the model developed for this dissertation. The Østbye et al. study does not use nationally representative data, therefore it is not known if the findings are an artifact of the population under study. The Thompson et al. (1998) study provides only aggregate estimates for US businesses, not individual-level estimates by weight status. The fuel consumption articles by Jacobsen and McLay, and Dannenberg do not provide individual-level estimates of excess fuel consumption by weight. Finally, only studies addressing costs of obesity in adults are included in this literature review, therefore the Trifiletti et al. study on child safety was also excluded.

	Country/ Topic Area	BMI Cutoffs	Study population / Methodology	Summary Results
ay mic on	United States / Automobile fuel consumption	None provided	Economic modeling	• 1988-2006: Annual consumption of extra of fuel due to increase in obesity lev • 1960 - 2006: Annual consumption of ext due to the increase in obesity levels. 0.7% of US annual fuel consumptio • Estimates 39 million gallons of gas for e in weight gained by the US auto pas

d	United States / Workers' compensation	Underweight: <18.5
		Normal: 18.5-24.9
		Overweight: 25-29.9
		Obese I: 30-34.9
		Obese II: 35-39.9
		Obese III: ≥ 40
			Retrospective cohort study - Duke Health and Safety Surveillance System. Subjects: 11,728 healthcare and university employees, 1997-2004	• Linear relationship between BMI and rat workdays, medical claims costs and costs
				• Lost workdays per 100 full-time equival normal, overweight, obese I, obese I
				  • 14.19, 60.17, 75.21, 117.61, 183.6:
				• Medical Claims Costs per 100 full-time (underweight, normal, overweight, obese III):
				  • $7109, $ 7503, $ 13,338, $19,661,
				• Indemnity claims costs per 100 full-time (underweight, normal, overweight, obese III):
				  • $3924, $5396, $13,569, $23,633, $

l f	United States / US business cost of life insurance and disability insurance	Normal: <25
		Mildly Obese: 25-28.9
		Moderately or Severely Obese: ≥ 29
			Population Attributable Risk. Data sources: National Health Interview Survey, Bureau of Labor Statistics and other agencies, published literature. Focused on employees aged 25-64	Diseases included: CHD, hypertension, type hypercholesterolemia, stroke, gall bladder d osteoarthritis, endometrial cancer
				• Aggregate obesity-attributable expenditur by US businesses:
				  • Life insurance: $1.8 billion
				  • Disability insurance: $800 million

Phase Two: Markov Model Results

Having reviewed the results of the obesity-related costing literature, this section presents the results of the Markov model and then provides a sensitivity analysis, which varies the model's assumptions in turn by CPI/discounting, BMI, starting age of cohort, race/ethnicity and gender, and finally, disability probability.

Baseline Results

The meta-analysis of the obesity-related costing literature clearly shows that external costs such as healthcare, absenteeism, productivity insurance and disability insurance are positively correlated with BMI $\geq$ 30. It has been argued however, that these costs may be negated by earlier mortality associated with higher weight levels. Results from the analysis conducted here suggest that this is not the case. **Given the costs, probabilities and other assumptions detailed in Chapter Three (which are likely conservative), the model developed for this dissertation calculates that the average lifetime, external cost of a person whose BMI is $\geq$30 at age 20 is \$54,579 (in \$2007) higher than a person whose starting BMI is 20. Approximately 9 million children are obese in the US. If all of these children remain obese at age 20, this would represent an external cost of approximately \$491 billion over their lifetimes.** The per-person external costs of obesity are shown in Table 4.6. The following section varies many of the model inputs in order to assess their effects on the overall costing. In no case, however, does the external, lifetime effect of obesity fall below zero, that is, that early mortality does not appear to mitigate lifetime costs of the obese on society.

Table 4.6: Lifetime Cost-Estimate of Obesity ($2007)

Lifetime Cost of Normal Weight 1000 Person Cohort	**Lifetime Cost of 1000 person Obese Cohort**	**Increased (Decreased) Cost of 1000 Person Cohort over Normal Weight Cohort**	**Average Increased (Decreased) Cost Per Person of Obese Cohort vs. Normal Weight Cohort**
$70,062,601	$124,641,872	**$54,579,271**	**$54,579**

Sensitivity Analysis

The results in Table 4.6 were based on the costs, probabilities and other assumptions that

are detailed in Chapter Three. However, it is often useful to alter these assumptions in

order to judge the sensitivity of the model's estimates. The model developed for this

dissertation was varied according to CPI/Discounting, BMI, starting age of the cohort,

and probability of receiving disability insurance. Results of the sensitivity analyses are

provided below.

CPI/Discounting

Table 4.7 displays the results of varying the CPI, discount, and MCPI rates on the

lifetime costs of obesity, holding other variables constant. The model's costing estimate

is sensitive to the discount rate used. If a discount rate of 3% is used, the average cost per

person increases to over $72,000 in 2007 dollars. If the discount rate is increased to 7%,

the average lifetime cost of obesity falls to just under $44,000. Altering the CPI and

MCPI rates do not appreciably alter the cost estimates, which range from approximately

$51,000 to over $62,000.

Table 4.7: Sensitivity Analysis of Lifetime Cost-Estimates of Obesity to CPI/Discounting ($2007)

Rate Change	Lifetime Cost of Normal Weight Cohort	Lifetime Cost of 1000 person Obese Cohort	Increased Cost of 1000 Person Cohort over Normal Weight Cohort	Average Increased Cost Per Person of Obese Cohort vs. Normal Weight Cohort
CPI 2%	$ 48,946,975	$ 99,912,629	$ 50,965,654	$ 50,966
CPI 4%	$121,070,548	$182,226,865	$ 61,156,317	$ 61,156
Discount Rate 3%	$174,901,632	$247,023,156	$ 72,121,524	$ 72,122
Discount Rate 7%	$ 28,896,323	$ 72,849,321	$ 43,952,998	$ 43,953
MCPI 3%	$ 70,062,601	$121,994,903	$ 51,932,302	$ 51,932
MCPI 5%	$ 70,062,601	$126,349,711	$ 56,287,110	$ 56,287
MCPI 6%	$ 70,062,601	$132,711,094	$ 62,648,493	$ 62,648

BMI

The BMI levels in the original 1000-person obese cohort were set to start at a range, in order to provide a more realistic representation of the 20 year-old, obese US population. It has been argued that increased mortality associated with higher BMI may negate other costs such as healthcare and absenteeism over a lifetime (Cawley, 2004). However, the sensitivity analysis performed on starting BMI displayed in Table 4.8 suggests this is not the case. The lifetime costs associated with obesity do appear sensitive to the effects of increasing BMI levels, ranging from $47,000 for BMI of 30, to over $91,000 for BMI of 45. Even at very high levels however, early mortality does not negate the costs associated with obesity. It appears that the costs of obesity rise quickly, particularly around BMI of 35, and while the incremental cost of obesity slows at BMI levels of 40 and above, at no point is it negative.

Table 4.8: Sensitivity Analysis of Lifetime Cost-Estimates of Obesity to BMI ($2007)

Starting BMI of Entire Obese Cohort	Lifetime Cost of 1000 person Obese Cohort	Lifetime Cost of Normal Weight Cohort (BMI of 20 at Start)	Increased Cost of 1000 Person Cohort over Normal Weight Cohort	Average Increased Cost Per Person of Obese Cohort vs. Normal Weight Cohort
BMI 30	$117,239,426	$70,062,601	$47,176,825	$47,179
BMI 32.5	$124,480,480	$70,062,601	$54,417,879	$54,418
BMI 35	$140,696,265	$70,062,601	$70,766,664	$70,767
BMI 37.7	$149,566,829	$70,062,601	$79,504,228	$79,504
BMI 40	$154,894,261	$70,062,601	$84,831,660	$84,832
BMI 42.5	$159,780,612	$70,062,601	$89,718,011	$89,718
BMI 45	$161,411,629	$70,062,601	$91,349,028	$91,349

Figure 4.1 charts the costs associated with the average external, lifetime costs of obesity by starting BMI. The chart shows that average costs rise swiftly with starting BMIs of 30 to 35. At BMIs above 40, average external costs appear to rise far more gradually. The Fontaine et al. (2003) lifetables do not provide information for BMIs above 45, but it appears that at starting BMI levels of above 45, external costs associated with obesity may indeed be negated by increased mortality.

Figure 4.1: Average Lifetime External Cost of Obese Cohort, Per Person, by BMI

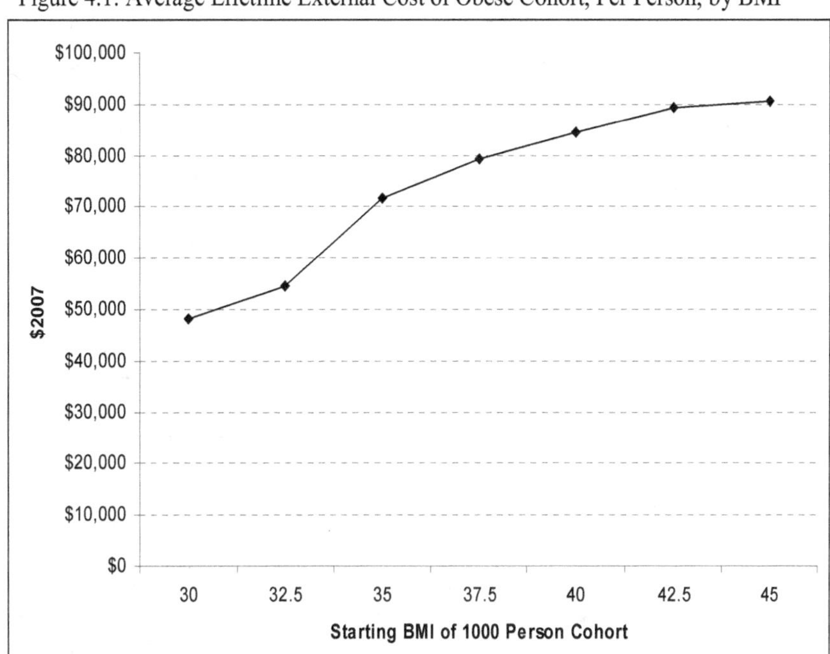

Starting Age of Cohort

It could be argued that starting the cohort analysis at age 20 may be unrealistic, although currently 17% of children 12-19 are obese (Ogden et al., 2006). Table 4.9 presents the effects of changing the starting age of the cohort to 40, from 20. This change does alter the lifetime costs, but not substantially ($54,500 to around $41,000).

Table 4.9: Sensitivity Analysis Lifetime Cost-Estimates of Obesity to Starting Age ($2007)

Starting Age of Cohort	Lifetime Cost of Normal Weight Cohort	Lifetime Cost of Obese Cohort	Increased Cost of 1000 Person Cohort over Normal Weight Cohort	Increased Cost Per Person of Obese Cohort vs. Normal Weight Cohort
20	$70,062,601	$124,641,872	**$54,579,271**	**$54,579**
40	$99,192,767	$139,934,893	**$40,742,126**	**$40,742**

The model does not appear sensitive to the increased probability estimates of social security disability insurance, as reported in Table 4.10. The model at baseline assumes increased incidence of disability at BMI of 30 of 10%, and 30% of BMI of 35 and above. If these probabilities are lowered to 5% and 10% respectively, the costs fall only very slightly, by approximately $700 per person. If the rates of disability are increased to 50% for BMI of 30-34.9 and 100% for BMIs equal or greater than 35, average lifetime costs approach $59,000, or around $4,000 per person greater than baseline.

Table 4.10: Sensitivity Analysis of Lifetime Cost-Estimates of Obesity to Disability ($2007)

	Lifetime Cost of Normal Weight Cohort	Lifetime Cost of 1000 Person Obese Cohort	Increased Cost of 1000 Person Cohort over Normal Weight Cohort	Increased Cost Per Person of Obese Cohort vs. Normal Weight Cohort
Increased SSDI Disability Risk:10%; 30% (Baseline)	$70,062,601	$124,641,872	**$54,579,271**	**$54,579**
Increased SSDI Disability Risk: 5%; 10%	$70,062,601	$123,997,400	**$53,934,799**	**$53,935**
Increased SSDI Disability Risk:25%; 50%	$70,062,601	$126,216,280	**$56,153,679**	**$56,154**
Increased SSDI Disability Risk:50%; 100%	$70,062,601	$128,911,249	**$58,848,648**	**$58,849**

Conclusion

The studies discussed in this chapter show that obesity is associated with increased costs in the following areas: healthcare, absenteeism, disability insurance, productivity and other costs. If the studies included different levels of obesity in their analyses, results tend to show a J-shaped relationship between obesity levels and these costs. Information contained in the meta-analysis of the obesity-related costing studies were used as inputs for development of the Markov model.

This Markov model of lifetime, external costs of obesity determined that on average, the lifetime, external cost of a 20-year old person with BMI $\geq$30 is almost $55,000 in 2007 dollars ($54,579) more than a person of normal weight over their lifetime (ages 20 to 85, or death). This amount is similar in range to the amount determined by economic modeling of lifetime, healthcare-related costs by Finkelstein et al. (2008), who calculated that healthcare costs for obese persons were $5,000 to $29,000 more than those of normal weight, depending on race, gender and obesity levels. The results of the Markov model developed here suggest that if all 9 million children in the United States became obese adults, it would represent an external cost of approximately $491 billion in $2007 in net present value over the course of their lifetimes. The next and final chapter provides a summary of this dissertation and discusses policy implications of these findings.

Chapter Five: Implications for Policy

Introduction

This dissertation examines increased obesity prevalence in the United States in the

context of market failure, and provides an answer to the research question: *What are the*

lifetime, external costs of obesity in the United States? It was previously thought

possible—from a purely economic lens—that shorter life expectancies due to increased

obesity rates, might mitigate the effects of direct and indirect costs associated with

obesity, such as healthcare and absenteeism (Cawley, 2007; Elston et al., 2007; Huchler

et al., 2005). In contrast, the results of the study presented here suggest that increased

obesity prevalence in the United States exacts substantial positive, lifetime, external

costs.

This chapter provides a summary of this dissertation and discusses the policy

implications of its findings. First, the chapter reviews and summarizes the background

on the issue of obesity; the obesity-related economic literature; the methodology of this

dissertation; and its results. Second, the evidence for obesity as market failure is

reviewed. Third, the implications for policy, and the types of options available to

policymakers to address increased obesity prevalence are presented. The chapter

concludes with a review of the limitations and contributions of the analysis presented

here.

Chapter One of this dissertation outlined the issue of increased obesity prevalence in the United States by detailing obesity trends and demographics, health and economic effects, and its correlates and causal influences. Obesity rates in the United States have risen dramatically in adults and children over the last 50 years, particularly since the early 1980s. Some racial and ethnic minority populations (e.g., African Americans, Native Americans and Mexican Americans) are disproportionately affected, however obesity levels have increased in all age and socio-demographic groups, and for both sexes.

Obesity increases mortality and is a risk factor for a wide range of diseases and other health conditions, including, but not limited to: cardiovascular disease, diabetes type 2, several forms of cancer, gallbladder disease, osteoarthritis, and depression. The science on the effects of obesity in childhood is still evolving, however, there are indications that the childhood effects of obesity may be even more deleterious on later health than obesity in adults. In addition, there also appear to be significant economic effects of increased obesity rates.

Individual biology and genetic makeup clearly contribute to overweight and obesity, yet individual differences such as these cannot explain such a rapid population-level increase in obesity rates over the last several decades. Instead, a myriad of environmental factors are implicated, including but not limited to: "micro-environmental" effects such as packaging, container size, and increased portion sizes; decreased walkability of neighborhoods; reduced access in some neighborhoods to affordable, nutritious food;

higher relative cost of healthier foods; increased technological advances that reduce requirements for physical activity; and food advertising to children. Many of these environmental variables may be modifiable by policy makers.

The review of the obesity-related economic literature in Chapter Two revealed that economists are divided on the issue of whether obesity represents an example of market failure. However, some economists argue that obesity represent examples of financial externalities, information failure and imperfect rationality. The literature review in Chapter Two also found that economic research on obesity falls into two main schools of thought: (1) Standard, or orthodox economics, and (2) behavioral economics. Research from standard, or neoclassical, economics may be divided into three main areas: costing; correlates and causal influences of obesity; and other analyses of specific phenomena, such as wage effects associated with obesity. There is also a small, but growing literature from behavioral economics, which questions basic assumptions about rationality regarding dietary behavior. Behavioral economics is a sub-field of economics informed by psychology, and assumes that human behavior departs from traditional economic assumptions of rationality in a predictable fashion.

The study presented was conducted in two phases, as detailed in Chapter Three: First, a meta-analysis of the costing literature related to obesity was undertaken. Second, a Markov model of lifetime, external costs was developed, using demographically representative, obese and normal weight 1000-person cohorts with TreeAge Pro 2009 Pro (TreeAge software, Williamstown, Massachusetts: www.treeage.com). The models developed used inputs located in the literature review and the meta-analysis of the obesity-related costing literature.

Chapter Four presented the results of this dissertation in its two phases. Phase One—the meta-analysis of the obesity-related costing literature—determined that costing literature related to obesity fell into five main categories: healthcare, absenteeism, disability and productivity and other analyses. In general, the obesity costing studies showed a "J-shaped" relationship between these costing areas and levels of obesity. That is, external costs were generally higher for the obese than for those of normal weight. In addition, external costs were often significantly higher for those in obesity classes II and III (BMI 35-39.9 and 40+) than for those in obesity category I. Phase Two of the study—development of the Markov model—found that a (likely conservative) estimate of the lifetime, external costs of an obese 1000-person cohort at age 20 was almost $55,000,000 in $2007 more than those of a cohort of those who were normal weight. If all 9 million obese children in the US become obese adults, this would represent a possible external cost of almost $500 billion over their lifetimes.

Having provided a brief summary of this dissertation's background, literature, methodology and results, the following section summarizes the literature relevant to the treatment of obesity as market failure, from economics, bio-medicine and public health.

According to standard welfare economics, government intervention is justified in the event of market failure. Therefore, establishment of market failure with regard to obesity is a critical first step with regard to government intervention, and policymaking. From the bio-medical, public health and economic literatures, and from the results of the study presented here, there appears to be evidence of three different kinds of market failures associated with obesity: (1) financial externalities; (2) information failure; and (3) imperfect rationality. These market failures are addressed in turn in the following sections.

Financial Externalities

Economists have been divided on the existence of financial and health externalities related to obesity. Increased healthcare costs due to treatment of obesity-related diseases had led to conjecture about the financial externalities (Anderson 2003b; Kuchler 2005; Cawley 2007; Elston 2007; McCormick 2007). However, because the lifetime, external costs had not been assessed, the existence of these externalities was speculative. Cawley (2004) even suggested the possibility for *positive* external effects on costs for the obese, given the shortened life expectancies linked with obesity.

A small number of studies have examined the lifetime costs associated with obesity (Allison et al., 1999; Finkelstein et al., 2008; Thompson et al., 1999; Tucker et al., 2006), but none in the context of lifetime, external costs for an obese versus normal weight cohort. Allison et al. assessed the aggregate lifetime costs of healthcare to the United

States. Thompson et al. looked at healthcare-related lifetime costs of in the United States. Tucker et al. examined internal costs, such as quality of life, as well as healthcare costs. Finkelstein et al. developed an economic model to estimate the lifetime costs of healthcare related to obesity for an obese versus normal weight cohort, and found that net, lifetime costs when accounting for weight-affected life expectancy suggested positive lifetime costs ranged from $5,340 to $29,460 in $2007, depending on race, gender and starting obesity levels. Further details on Finkelstein et al.'s study are provided in Table 4.1.

In contrast, this dissertation developed an estimate of healthcare and other external costs, which also included absenteeism, disability, productivity and wage effects (foregone taxes). The findings reported here support the existence of significant financial externalities (approximately $55,000 in $2007 per person over his or her lifetime) associated with obesity in the United States. If all 9 million obese children in the United States became obese adults, that would represent external costs of $497 Billion. The findings of this dissertation and those of Finkelstein et al. (2008), suggest that increased obesity levels result in significant financial externalities.

Information Failure

Although evidence is mixed, there is also some support for information failure in the context of obesity, particularly in the area of under-provision of information. As described in Chapter Two, Cawley (2004) described information regarding diet and physical activity as "underprovided and disseminated" by governments, in comparison to the provision of information by food and beverage manufacturers. In this case, it may be costly for consumers to source and use appropriate diet and physical activity-related information. It is also possible that people may be unaware of the nutritional content of the food they consume. Nutrition labels on packaged foods provide calorie and other macronutrient information, but this information is generally not accessible in food consumed away from home. Further, studies show that average intake of food away from home has increased (Binkley, 2006). It is also possible that Americans may not be aware of their own personal risk, although this is disputed by Finkelstein (2008). Kuchler et al. (2005) note that in one study, 41 percent of people who were overweight did not perceive themselves as such and 13 percent of people whose BMI was equal to or greater than 30 perceived their weight as low to normal.

Imperfect Rationality

The literature relevant to the economic concept of rationality as an example of market failure may be divided into that associated with children and that in adults. In children, it is well accepted in economics that children are not rational actors and cannot accurately judge their own welfare (McCormick et al., 2007). As described in Chapter Two, several economists have noted that lack of rationality in children represents an example of market failure in the context of obesity (Anderson et al., 2003b; Cawley 2004; Moodie et al., 2006; McCormick et al., 2007).

In adults, many neoclassical economists assume fully rational behavior with regard to diet and physical activity behavior (Cawley, 2007; Finkelstein and Zuckerman, 2008;

Philipson and Poser, 2001. As Philipson noted: "More than many physical conditions, obesity is avoidable by behavioral changes, which economists expect to be undertaken if the benefits exceed the costs… In a rational-choice model… there is no such thing as 'overweight'. Weight is the result of personal choices along such dimensions as occupation , leisure-time activity or inactivity, residence, and, of course, food intake" (p.1). Behavioral economists however, allow for imperfect rationality: "Behavioral economists have found that individuals tend to deviate from what is often termed rational behavior in highly systematic and predictable ways" (Just, 2006, p.210).

Evidence from public health literature suggests that at least some dietary behavior in adults may not be fully rational in the economic sense, and may be unreflective and subconscious. As discussed in Chapter One, Wansink and colleagues have found evidence of many contextual effects on eating behavior (Wansink & Kim, 2005a; Wanksink et al., 2005b; Wansink, 2006; Wansink et al., 2007a, 2007c; Wansink & Van Ittersum, 2007b). In experiments such as those with nutritionists and ice-cream, movie-goers with popcorn, and diners with a refillable soup bowls, Wansink and colleagues have found many instances of micro-environmental effects on individual consumption. Further, the results of these experiments suggest that the individuals under study were often completely unaware of these effects. Examples of these micro-environmental effects include: the size of the container from which one consumes foods or beverages; the context (e.g., in a movie theatre); and casual mentioning of the state of origin of a bottle of wine. Also mentioned in Chapter One, Christakis and Fowler (2007) studied the effect of social networks on weight gain, and found that independent of geography or blood relationship, if a spouse, friend or relative of an individual gained or lost weight, it predicted weight gain or loss in that individual. If one was making (economically) rational decisions regarding consumption of food and beverages, then subconscious cues such as portion size, and the weight gain or loss of friends or relatives should not affect dietary behavior or BMI.

Finally, there is limited evidence in bio-medical literature that for some people certain foods or macronutrients may be addictive (Avena, Rada, & Hoebel, 2008; Spring et al., 2008; Yanovski, 2003). The tobacco control literature on addiction suggests that addiction may also be evidence of imperfect rationality (Chaloupka, Tauras, & Grossman, 2000; Jha, Musgrove, Chaloupka, & Yurekli, 2001).

Therefore, it seems that increased rates of obesity in the United States may represent examples of the market failures of financial externalities, information failure, and imperfect rationality (certainly in children and possibly in adults). The present study provides evidence of financial externalities; further research on information failure and imperfect rationality is needed. The following section discusses the public policy implications and policy options of these findings.

Implications for Policy

The findings of the analysis conducted for this dissertation, in addition to the economic, bio-medical and public health literatures, suggest that increased obesity prevalence may represent examples of financial externalities, information failure, and imperfect rationality. The findings of the analysis presented here and that of other researchers

suggest that the financial externalities of obesity are significant. These findings in turn,

suggest that government intervention is warranted. An important first question before

intervening, however, is whether the issue is remediable, i.e., whether policymakers may

adequately redress the situation. Although there are basic biological and genetic

differences that account for weight differences, it is unlikely that the rise in obesity

prevalence in the population in the last several decades can be attributed to genetics and

biology alone. Rather, many environmental changes throughout the socio-ecological

model, described in Chapter One, are implicated in changing dietary and physical activity

behavior. Several of these environmental variables may be manipulated by policymakers.

Therefore, it would seem that increased obesity prevalence may indeed be remediable by

policymakers.

The specifics and effectiveness of policy interventions to address obesity rates remain a

question, however. There have been many successful policy interventions in public

health, e.g., vaccinations, seatbelts, and tobacco control (Homer & Simson, 2007;

Hopkins et al., 2001; Lake & Townshend, 2006). Many have drawn parallels between

tobacco control and efforts to address obesity (Chopra & Darnton-Hill, 2004; Mercer et

al., 2003; Yach, McKee, Lopez, & Novotny, 2005). However, there are key differences in

the targeted behavior change associated with smoking, and with that of diet and physical

activity. There are no safe levels of tobacco consumption, and the behavior change

sought by public health officials is to cease, or never start, smoking. In contrast, the

change required in dietary behavior of many in the United States is nuanced. Food is required for human life, which is not the case for tobacco. The dietary change needed by many Americans is to reduce consumption of solid fats, added sugars, and refined flour, while increasing consumption of fruit, vegetables, whole grains, legumes, and lean protein (DHHS and USDA, 2005). Unlike smoking, physical activity is a behavior that policy makers would like to encourage, rather than prevent. The following section outlines the types of policies that could potentially address the market failures associated with obesity.

Policy Options

This section provides a selection of policy options—and the market failures they seek to address—that might be undertaken by policymakers at different levels of government. Several of these policies are already being implemented. There are promising results from programs intended to reduce obesity rates, particularly some targeting children in schools (see, for instance Economos et al., 2007). However, knowledge regarding the effectiveness of many federal, state and local policies intended to reduce obesity prevalence—particularly among adults—is still relatively limited.

Given the large number of environmental variables implicated in obesity's rise, and the tools available to policymakers at different levels of government, such as taxes, regulations, subsidies, information campaigns (Salamon, 2002), there may be an infinite number of policies to reduce obesity rates. Therefore, this section is intended to be illustrative only of the policies that could be, or are being, implemented; a comprehensive catalog of policy options to address obesity is beyond the scope of this dissertation. The policy options described here are broken into those that are intended to address obesity in (1) children and (2) adults. The market failures associated with obesity may help inform policy choices. It is important to note, however, that policy options to reduce obesity rates need not necessarily target a particular market failure. Examples of policy options to address obesity in children and adults are described in the section that follows, following a brief discussion of the potential role of taxes.

A Note on Taxes

Taxes are often used as corrective measures when consumers do not bear the full costs of their consumption decisions (Cordes, 2002; Grossman, Sindelar, Mullahy, & Anderson, 1993), and have been mentioned as an option for policymakers in combating obesity (Chriqui, Eidson, Bates, Kowalczyk & Chaloupka, 2008; Jacobson & Brownell, 2000). However, implementing taxes on food products or components such as fat or sugar may be problematic for a number of reasons. First, operationalization of such a tax may be extremely complex. Taxing a category of food (e.g., "junk food") would require careful definition of this food classification, with inevitable loopholes. Taxing an ingredient (e.g., fat or sugar) is likely to be far more complicated than taxing a particular kind of food, and could cause further complications by the distinctions required in the case of fats between those that are considered "good" (i.e., mono- and poly-saturated) and "bad" (i.e., saturated and *trans*-) fats. Secondly, there may be unanticipated consequences of a tax, such as substitution effects. For example, taxing fat may cause the population to increase sugar consumption, or vice versa. A tax on sugar-sweetened soda may be easier to justify and implement than taxes on certain food groups or macro-nutrients. First, the product may be identified and differentiated relatively easily. Second, sugar-sweetened soda

provides only trace nutritional benefit in addition to simple calories. Third, there is good,

scientific evidence of the negative impact of sugar-sweetened soda on weight and health

(Ebbeling et al., 2006; Ludwig, Petersen, & Gortmaker, 2001; Malik, Schulze, & Hu,

2006; Schulze et al., 2004).

Policy Options: Children

Market failures associated with obesity in children include financial externalities and

imperfect rationality. It is accepted that children are not rational actors (McCormick et

al., 2007), and basic human biology provides preferences for sweet and salty tastes (Birch

& Fisher, 1998). In addition, the older the child when he or she is obese, the more likely

they are to become an obese adult (Guo & Chumlea, 1999). Examples of policies related

to obesity in children include regulating food and physical activity environments in

schools, and food advertising to children, described below.

Regulation of School Food and Physical Activity Environments

There are several potential arguments for regulation of the food and physical activity

environments in the nation's schools. First, policymakers have clear jurisdiction in

schools. Second, children reportedly consume 19-50% of their daily calories at school

(Burghardt et al., 1993), and competitive foods have been shown to displace fruit and

vegetables (Kubik et al., 2003). Third, a relatively small change in consumption over

time (80 to 250 calories per day) seems to have led to the rise in obesity in children

(Koplan et al., 2005).Therefore, a similarly small change may have the desired effect of reducing obesity levels in children.

Several initiatives have been developed at local and state levels to modify the food environment in schools. One example is in California, which regulates competitive foods (food that is not part of the breakfast and school lunch programs) that may be sold in elementary, middle and high schools. California State Senate Bills 12 and 985 passed the California legislature in 2005 and came into effect in 2007 (California Department of Education, 2008a, 2008b). These laws regulate the amount of fat, total calories and sugar in foods and sweeteners in beverages, among other things, in competitive foods that may be sold in California schools (California Education Code Sections 49430-49431.7). At least 15 other states have implemented nutrition requirements for competitive foods in schools (Trust for America's Health, 2005, 2006).

Policymakers may also increase physical education (PE) requirements for children and teens as a way to reduce incidence and prevalence of obesity in these populations. According to researchers, children and teens attended daily PE classes in 3.8%, 7.8% and 2.1% of elementary, middle and high schools respectively (Lee, Burgeson, Fulton, & Spain, 2007). Research by Burgeson et al., (2001) showed that slightly more than 50% of students in elementary school were required to participate in physical education, but this fell sharply in middle school and high school to 5.4% for grade 12. Using objective measures, Troiano et al. (2008) found that 42% of children in the US aged 6-11 get the recommended 60 minutes of daily physical activity, compared to only 8% of teens.

Another option available to policymakers to reduce obesity levels in children may be to regulate food advertising to children. A report by the IOM found evidence that food advertising to children influences their food-related requests, preferences and consumption (McGinnis et al., 2005). Further, children under the age of eight cannot distinguish the persuasive intent of advertising, and children under the age of four cannot differentiate between advertising and programming (McGinnis et al., 2005). A recent paper by Chou, Rashad and Grossman (2008) calculated that removing the tax deduction for businesses associated with food advertising to children and teens would reduce obesity levels in those populations by 5 to 7%. This same study forecast that a complete ban on marketing of unhealthy food to children and teens would reduce obesity in children 3-11 by 18%, and in teens 12-18 by 14%.

Policy Options: Adults

Possible market failures associated with obesity in adults include financial externalities, information failure and imperfect rationality. However, because there is the possibility that adults may be fully informed and acting rationally, and given the lack of a specific forum—such as schools—for change, the policy options available are different to those available for children. In reducing obesity rates in adults, the work on libertarian paternalism by Thaler and Sunstein (2003, 2008) and others, such as O'Donohue and Rabin (2003) may be informative. Libertarian paternalism draws from behavioral economics in its understanding of human behavior and rationality, and seeks to "nudge" people in a direction that they would acknowledge is in their best interests, but allows them to act against these interests should they wish to do so. O'Donoghue and Rabin (2003) suggest looking for the most feasible policies that are minimally interventionist and help people who may not be acting in a fully rational manner, but not penalize people who are. Examples of these policies include education, alterations to short-term incentives and easily modified default choices (O'Donohue and Rabin (2003).

Table 5.1 displays illustrative policies in keeping with a libertarian paternalistic philosophy. These examples represent a variety of policy areas and different levels of government and are marked by the market failure they are intended to address. The large number of environmental variables implicated in the rise of obesity levels suggests that many policy interventions may be necessary. The successful public health efforts to reduce tobacco use may be instructive. The strategies used to reduce tobacco consumption included the combination of clinical interventions, education, regulation, and economic incentives (Mercer et al., 2003).

It is only recently that policies have been implemented to address obesity. To date there is little evidence of the effectiveness or otherwise of proposed or implemented policies in adults. Evaluation of "natural experiments" or public policies intended to reduce obesity prevalence will be important to inform policymaking with regard to obesity.

Please note that many of the policies in the cells of Table 5.1 table may be undertaken by multiple levels of government; the table is intended to show the wide number of possible policy interventions, not that these policies can only be actions by that specific level of government. The policy areas in the table—food, agriculture and trade; healthcare; transportation and community planning; and the information environment—derive from a report of a meeting convened in 2007 by the National Cancer Institute on defining an obesity policy research agenda (McKinnon et al., 2009). The sections that follow discuss each of the policies by policy area.

Table 5.1: Examples of Policy Options to Address Obesity in Adults

Policy Area / Gov't Level	Food, Agriculture, Trade	Healthcare	Transportation, Community Planning	Information Environment, e.g., Media
Federal	Changes to WIC* and SNAP† Benefit Programs (R)	Medicare reimbursement for obesity counseling (I, R)	Subsidies for cycle commuting (2008 TARP bill) (R)	Whole package calorie labeling (I)
State	Tax on sweetened beverages (F)	Medicaid reimbursement for obesity counseling (R)	Infrastructure for "active transportation" (walking, cycling) (R)	Informational campaigns targeting high risk groups (I)
Local (city, county)	Calorie Labeling in Restaurants (R)	-	Zoning (R)	Point of decision prompts (R)

*WIC = Special Supplemental Nutrition Program for Women Infants and Children;
†SNAP = Supplemental Nutrition Assistance Program (formerly known as Food Stamp benefits)
Market Failure Targets: F=Financial Externality; I=Information; R=Rationality

Food, Agriculture and Trade

WIC: Following a report by the IOM (2006), the Special Supplemental Nutrition Program for Women, Infants and Children (WIC) was modified to encourage breastfeeding among program participants and to expand the list of foods and beverages required by participating WIC-authorized stores and available to WIC beneficiaries (Food and Nutrition Service [FNS] , 2007). This program will be fully implemented in October 2009 (FNS, 2008). Foods and beverages available for purchase to WIC participants have been expanded to include soy beverages, legumes, canned fish (such as sardines, salmon and tuna), and fruits and vegetables (FNS, 2007). These changes to WIC may also expand healthy food choices for non-WIC beneficiaries. This policy change may address the market failure associated with rationality by reducing costs associated with improved diet.

<u>SNAP Program:</u> The Food, Conservation and Energy Act of 2008, P.L. 110-246, (a.k.a the 2008 "Farm Bill") renamed the Food Stamp Program the "Supplemental Nutrition Assistance Program" (SNAP), and authorized the USDA to conduct a pilot of study of incentives for SNAP beneficiaries to consume healthier diets. This follows a report by the GAO on the feasibility of the program for this purpose (Government Accountability Office [GAO], 2008). This policy change may address the market failure associated with rationality by reducing costs associated with improved diet.

<u>"Junk Food" Tax for Medicaid funding or other Health Measures:</u> Many states in the United States have imposed small taxes on snack foods or soft drinks, with revenue raised from the taxes often going to general state funds (Chriqui, Eidson, Bates, Kowalczyk & Chaloupka, 2008; Jacobson & Brownell, 2000). These small taxes could be used instead to raise revenue for health promotion measures, or for healthcare services, such as Medicaid. New York State has recently announced its intention to implement an "obesity tax" of 18% on sugared soft drinks, which is expected to raise $404 million in revenue (Chan, 2008; Paterson, 2008). Such a policy may address the market failures associated with the financial externalities of obesity, and rationality, by providing increased immediate costs.

Calorie Labeling in Restaurants: In 2007, New York City introduced regulations that required calorie information to be posted in restaurants with more than 15 outlets in the US (McColl, 2008). Calorie labeling regulations are now under consideration in 20 cities and states in the US (McColl, 2008). As mentioned in Chapter One, the frequency with which people consume food away from home has increased over the last several decades (Guthrie, Lin, & Frazao, 2002). Research has also shown that many consumers underestimate the number of calories available in fast food restaurant meals (Burton, Creyer, Kees, & Huggins, 2006), and that calorie information in many restaurants in New York City was often not readily available to consumers (Bassett et al., 2008). According to a study conducted in 2007, if calorie information was seen, consumers chose menu items with fewer calories (Bassett et al., 2008). Rigorous evaluation of the effectiveness of calorie labeling regulations is needed. Such a regulation provides information for consumers when making food and beverage purchasing decisions at the point of purchase, and addresses potential information failure.

Healthcare

Medicare and Medicaid Reimbursement for Obesity Counseling: Reimbursement for obesity screening and treatment could be provided by Medicare and Medicaid. Medicare currently provides preventive treatment services for enrollees (Centers for Medicare and Medicaid Services [CMS], 2007). Patients are reimbursed for a variety of preventive services, such as colonoscopies, mammograms, flu shots, and tobacco cessation counseling (CMS, 2007). However, similar services for obesity are not currently available. In 1996, the US Preventive Services Task Force associated with the Agency for

Healthcare Research and Quality (AHRQ) recommended screening for obesity in adults by physicians, and the provision of diet and/or physical activity-related intensive counseling and behavioral interventions (U.S. Preventive Services Task Force, 1996). This counseling and intervention work produced sustained weight loss of 3-5kg and improved other markers such as blood pressure and glucose metabolism (U.S. Preventive Services Task Force, 2003). This policy intervention may address the market failures of obesity associated with information failure and rationality.

Transportation and Community Planning

<u>Fringe Benefits for Bicycle Commuting:</u> The Emergency Economic Stabilization Act of 2008 adds bicycle commuting to the list of fringe benefits that may be provided by employers to workers. From January 1 2009, employees may be reimbursed to $20 per month from employers if they commute to work by bicycle. The benefit may be used to reimburse improvements to bicycles, or their repair and storage (Public Law 110-343, Div. B, Act Sec 211(a)). Such a regulation provides proximal (monetary) incentives, rather than the distal benefits of improved health, for increased physical activity, and may address the market failure associated with imperfect rationality, and the human tendency to discount future benefits for immediate rewards.

<u>Infrastructure for "Active Transportation":</u> "Active transportation" or "active commuting" involves walking or cycling to and from work. It may be appropriate for state governments (as well as federal and local governments) to provide funding and incentives to increase walking and cycling for transit in the population. A study of young

adults showed that active transportation was inversely associated with weight (Gordon-Larsen, Nelson, & Beam, 2005), and other research suggests that active commuting is a method to increase physical activity adherence (Berrigan, Troiano, McNeel, DiSogra, & Ballard-Barbash, 2006). Examples of policies to increase active commuting may include funding for traffic-calming measures (such as speed bumps or reduced speed limits), and/or infrastructure such as bike lines, mixed-use trails, and wide sidewalks. As an example of policy to provide incentives for active commuting, the state government of Western Australia recently implemented a "pedestrian-friendly subdivision design code", and residents' walking for transportation increased relative to residents of another community who acted as controls (Giles-Corti et al., 2008). Policies to increase walking and cycling for transit would address the market failures associated with rationality by reducing the immediate costs to individuals of increased physical activity.

Urban Planning and Development: Research suggests that local governments may facilitate increased physical activity in the population through changes in urban planning and design (Frank & Kavage, 2008: Giles-Corti et al., 2008; Handy, Cao, & Mokhtarian, 2008; Saelens & Handy, 2008). Over one hundred years ago, urban planning rules and regulations were created in response to often unhealthy inner-city environments, which lead to the separation of employment and residence, and urban sprawl that required cars for transportation (Frank & Kavage, 2008). A recent review of the literature regarding the built environment and physical activity found that several characteristics of urban environments are associated with increased physical activity of residents, including: distance to destinations, mixed land use (combining retail, employment and residential areas) and density (Saelens & Handy, 2008). Saelens and Handy list two important ways in which local governments may increase physical activity of residents: land use patterns (e.g., mixed land use) and transportation systems (e.g., traffic-calming measures, widening sidewalks, increased street connectivity). Frank and Kavage (2008) note that implementing "grid" street designs enable activity, rather than the familiar cul-de-sac residential areas that require automobile transportation to destinations such as school, shops and employment. Physical activity-friendly local government policies may address the market failure associated with rationality by reducing costs to activity.

Information Environment

<u>Whole Package Calorie Labeling</u>: In 1994, the Food and Drug Administration (FDA) updated the Nutrition Labeling and Education Act (NLEA) (Silverglade, 1996), which requires that most food packages provide information on calories as well as on certain micro and macronutrients—such as iron, calcium and protein—in a standardized form. Research suggests that this information is used by many consumers at least some of the time (Cowburn & Stockley, 2005), and that this information in turn affects dietary outcomes (Variyam, 2008; Variyam & Cawley, 2006). Under the current NLEA, calorie information is provided in a "per serving" format, in addition to the number of servings contained in the packaging. Yet research shows that many consumers, particularly those who are older, and/or low SES, have difficulty calculating the caloric value for the whole package (Cowburn & Stockley, 2005). Adding "whole package calorie information" to the nutritional information provided on food may increase awareness of the total caloric

value of a package of food among consumers. This initiative may address the obesity-related market failure associated with information failure.

Informational Campaigns Targeting High Risk Groups: State or other governments may increase funding for informational campaigns on the importance attaining/maintaining a healthy weight, healthy eating, and regular physical activity among targeted groups at higher risk for obesity. Behavioral economics and psychology suggest that humans like to conform (Thaler & Sunstein, 2008), therefore an information campaign, which includes prominent members of the target community engaging in physical activity and/or healthy eating, may be effective. This policy intervention may address the market failure associated with information failure and rationality.

Point-of-Decision Prompts: Point-of-decision prompts, which encourage physical activity rather than mechanized alternatives in the population, (e.g., stair use instead of escalators), may be a method for local governments to increase population physical activity. These prompts often take the form of motivational signs that provide health benefit reminders to the public at the "point of decision", when individuals are presented with the option to take the stairs or the escalator, e.g., "Save time, keep your heart healthy, use the stairs" (Russell & Hutchinson, 2000). These prompts have been implemented in diverse public settings, including airports, train stations and shopping centers (Dolan et al., 2006). A review article by Dolan et al. (2006) reported that point of decision prompts increased stair use by 2.8%. These policy interventions may address the market failure associated with imperfect rationality.

Having reviewed a few of the many options available to policymakers to reduce obesity prevalence, the following section discusses the limitations and contributions of the analysis of this dissertation.

Limitations and Contributions

This study presented here is limited in several ways. First, published sources were used to determine the costing inputs and categories for the Markov model described in Chapters Three and Four. However, primary analysis to determine these costs and categories was beyond the scope of this particular study. In addition, published costing studies were rigorously reviewed to determine costing inputs. Second, it is likely that not all costing inputs were included. For instance, the study presented here assessed costs for a single generation of the 1000 person cohorts. Given the effects of maternal obesity on children, it is likely that there are multi-generational costs associated with obesity that were not captured in the results presented here. In addition, the studies that are summarized in Table 4.5 suggest that other societal costs of obesity may exist, but these costs were not included in the present analysis for the reasons noted in Chapter Four. However, the likelihood that not all costs were included in the model developed here suggests that the final calculations are conservative.

Third, the demographic make-up of the cohorts developed for the lifetime costing model may not adequately represent the United States population. Only non-Hispanic whites, non-Hispanic blacks and Hispanics were included in the cohorts of the model developed for this dissertation, omitting other racial and ethnic minority groups. In addition, the study assumes that the obesity figures for Mexican Americans are representative for Hispanics in the United States. Given that the majority of Hispanics in the United States are Mexican Americans, and the high prevalence of obesity in Mexican Americans, their inclusion in the model as detailed in Chapter Three appears reasonable, and superior to the alternative of omitting Hispanics from the model altogether. Finally, the results of the Markov model are a projection, not a prediction. It may be that medical breakthroughs might lead to effective treatment of obesity, which is not accounted for in the model. Nevertheless, the model developed here provides a method of assessing lifetime, external costs of obesity, based on the best available evidence.

Despite these limitations, the study presented here makes a number of contributions to the literature on policy and obesity. First, this study appears to be the first rigorous estimate of the lifetime, external costs of obesity, and provides an answer to the question in economic literature regarding whether obesity-related lifetime, external costs are positive or negative. The finding that the lifetime external costs of obesity appear to be net positive is significant, provides evidence of financial externalities, and suggests that policy intervention to reduce obesity incidence and prevalence is warranted. Second, the present study provides a rigorous review and summary of the obesity-related healthcare costing literature

Third, the basic structure of the model developed for this dissertation is the first obesity-costing model to be developed that is demographically representative of the United States, for which the starting BMI of the cohort is a range, and that varies BMI throughout the "life" of the cohort. Other researchers may use, alter or build upon the basic model structure developed here for future costing analyses.

Fourth, other cohort-based models of obesity-related lifetime costs (e.g., Finkelstein et al., 2008, and Tucker et al., 2006) provide results for race/gender-specific cohorts. The model described here is as demographically representative of the United States as possible given data constraints, and thus provides results relevant to obesity in the US population overall, rather than the costs associated with racial and gender-based sub-populations. Providing results at the sub-population level may suggest to some that it is more or less important to intervene in some demographic groups, when the underlying cohort cost disparities may simply reflect social inequities, such lack of access to healthcare.

Finally, this dissertation summarizes economic literature on the market failures associated with widespread obesity at the population level, and finds support in the economic and public health literature for market failures associated with financial externalities, information failure and imperfect rationality. Overall, the study presented here should aid understanding of the social costs of widespread and increasing levels of obesity.

Conclusion

Obesity rates have risen substantially for children and adults in the United States over the last several decades, with serious health and economic consequences. Using inputs derived from a structured literature search and other authoritative sources, this dissertation developed a model that calculated the net present value of the lifetime, external costs of obesity. The present study found that the average, lifetime, external costs of an obese person is approximately $55,000 more than someone of normal weight in $2007. If all 9 million obese children in the United States become obese adults, this would represent a combined external cost of $491 billion in $2007. Further, these estimates may be conservative. Results from the literature and the model developed for this study suggest that the market failures associated with increased obesity prevalence include: financial externalities, information failure and imperfect rationality.

For children, examples of policies to reduce or prevent obesity include regulation of school food and physical activity environments, and food marketing to children. In adults, policies that align with a libertarian paternalistic approach may be effective. Examples of policies that target obesity in adults include encouraging active transportation, mixed use zoning and calorie labeling in restaurants. Although there are promising results from interventions targeting children, little is currently known about the effectiveness of policy options at federal, state and local levels for adults. Careful, rigorous evaluation of policy interventions will be important.

Rising obesity levels will exact serious financial and human costs. Government intervention to reduce obesity incidence and prevalence appears warranted.